T0093696

Empathy, Normalization and De-escalation

Massimo Biondi • Massimo Pasquini
Lorenzo Tarsitani

Editors

Empathy, Normalization and De-escalation

Management of the Agitated Patient in Emergency and Critical Situations

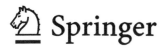 Springer

Editors
Massimo Biondi
Department of Human Neurosciences
Sapienza University of Rome
Rome
Italy

Massimo Pasquini
Department of Human Neuroscience
Sapienza University of Rome
Rome
Italy

Lorenzo Tarsitani
Department of Human Neurosciences
Sapienza University of Rome
Rome
Italy

ISBN 978-3-030-65105-3   ISBN 978-3-030-65106-0   (eBook)
https://doi.org/10.1007/978-3-030-65106-0

This Springer imprint is published by the registered company Springer Nature Switzerland AG
The registered company address is: Gewerbestrasse 11, 6330 Cham, Switzerland

Preface

Introduction: Meaning of the END Methods

Understanding social relations and the complexity of human behaviors in interpersonal relationships is really challenging. In this book we aimed to provide a full presentation of the main techniques and the practical skills to manage an agitated person in clinical and nonclinical settings. Working for several years in a psychiatric intensive care unit (PICU) as well as in an Emergency Department of one of the largest hospital in Italy, in the downtown of Rome, we have experienced everyday clinical situations of managing aggressive and potentially violent people. Later we introduced an easy and practical course for medical and paramedical staff for more than 10 years now. We also have learned that specific skills such as be calm, empathic, and de-escalate agitated persons are in some ways innate for somebody, while they are not innate for others. On the other hand clinicians found out very useful and innovative ways to learn communication techniques in hard situations. Talking to a scared or aggressive person is difficult, but this ability could be learnt.

It is constituted by two distinctive parts: the knowledge component, which regards theory and the primary nonverbal and verbal communication skills, and the practical component, which is to do with the ability to choose the right words at the right time with the right tone with the pivotal respect of listening to what the person is talking about without judgment. When a healthcare professional assists an aggressive patient the main rules are: to be calm and to work safety. Only successively the several techniques of de-escalation and normalization could be applied.

When we ask ourselves if we are emphatic in general or if we are more empathic in certain situation different sets of answers are possible. Apart from personal attitudes, many factors influence this feeling: the sense of belonging to a proper contest, the sense of place, and more ethnical, political, or professional identity. Even if nonverbal communication represents the most important issue in this kind of situations, language is pivotal. In our experience it is more simple to de-escalate a person when we share with her/him the same slang. This is because we reciprocally recognize our origins. At the opposite even if you are well experienced in managing agitated person it doesn't come so natural to think ourselves doing the same in a culturally diverse country. Nonverbal posturing and linguistic barriers may alter our skills. While some de-escalating and normalization procedures can be considered universally recognized. The END method consists in three main components:

Empathy, Normalization, and De-escalation. It is a sequence and every component has a theoretical background and practical norms to act.

The rationale is based on the ability to manage feelings, thoughts, and manifested behaviors in order to prevent aggression and violence, but also to build up a therapeutic alliance in several settings, and to reduce the forced hospitalizations. Our thinking as authors derived from our experience as psychiatrist but also from the experience of teaching these concepts to hundreds of colleagues. As editors we have retained the virtue of keeping these abilities simple. This is due to the decision to report what happens in clinical settings.

We start with a chapter focused on the definition of psychomotor agitation and aggression. Aggressiveness can be expressed verbally or behaviorally, and different levels of intention and consciousness may characterize specific conditions and behaviors. During the first END course it was astonishing to find out how many colleagues were familiar with these definitions. The nature of these conditions will be fully discussed.

Whereas in Chap. 3 readers find a very thorough review of the neurobiology of aggression and violence, the ability to modulate our own empathy in certain conditions is stated in Chap. 4.

It is not so obvious to psychologists and psychiatrists when, why, and with which person we have to be less or more empathetic. Many colleagues have served this incompetence. In everyday clinical activities unconsciously we normalize certain situations, besides a comprehensive description of the former technique is explored in Chap. 5.

The core issue of how to de-escalate an agitated person is fully presented in Chap. 6. Here readers will find out a set of techniques and guidelines in order to improve prevention and reduce damage risk for patients, healthcare operators, and family members who can often be victims of violence. De-escalation is conceived as part of the process of managing aggression and it is considered both as a preventive measure and the most reliable technique to avoid violent outbreaks deterioration. In Chap. 7 the safer and widely used protocol of pharmacological interventions for the agitated person is fully illustrated. Thus, an effective communication is central in patient's comprehension of treatment benefits and risks and increases compliance. A risk of impaired capacity to consent to treatment has often been associated with specific clinical characteristics, among these are excitement and positive symptoms together with psychiatric symptoms' severity, cognitive dysfunction, and impaired executive functioning. For these reasons in Chap. 8 authors describe how a good and supportive doctor–patient communication and a valid informed consent acquisition are often hindered by several issues, among which the clinician's fear of hurting the patient by communicating a bad diagnosis or not knowing how to manage the patient's emotional reactions. Finally, the relevance of a post-aggression debrief will be discussed for its role as a way to give significance to aggressive events in terms of possible shared meaning between the patient and the staff. In other words, debriefing will be presented as a chance to comprehend the patient's psychopathological world, to restore a narrative coherence beyond the traumatic and violent event, and to keep a safe and trustable therapeutic environment.

Rome, Italy   Massimo Biondi
                                                                                    Massimo Pasquini
                                                                                     Lorenzo Tarsitani

Contents

Psychomotor Agitation and Aggression

1

Federico Dazzi, Martina Valentini, and Lorenzo Tarsitani

1.1 Introduction and Definition

Consistently with our approach [1], in a dimensional perspective, agitation and aggression represent the behavioral expression of two psychological dimensions: activation and aggressiveness. Indeed, according to the definitions and anchor points provided by Pancheri et al. [2] for the Rapid Dimensional Assessment Scale (RADAS or SVARAD, the acronym in Italian), an instrument aimed to rapidly assess some basic psychopathological dimensions, the anger/aggressiveness dimension may include verbal or physical violence, whether activation is characterized by increased motor and psychological activity, which are hallmarks of psychomotor agitation.

Activation and aggressiveness can be best conceptualized as psychopathological dimensions rather than symptoms or disorders, as they fall on a continuum ranging from normal and physiological functions to psychopathological conditions; they are not the expression of specific disorders, but they are rather transdiagnostic; at least in part, they share underlying neurobiological patterns. According to these characteristics, in a dimensional perspective, they can be better conceptualized as distinct constructs. Though both literature and clinical experience support such distinction, the boundaries between activation and aggressiveness, and even more between their clinical expression, are not always clear, and they frequently overlap. Before going

F. Dazzi (✉)
Department of Human Sciences, LUMSA University, Rome, Italy

M. Valentini
Department of Human Neurosciences, Sapienza University of Rome, Rome, Italy
e-mail: martina.valentini@uniroma1.it

L. Tarsitani
Department of Neurosciences and Mental Health, Policlinico Umberto I Hospital, Sapienza University of Rome, Rome, Italy
e-mail: lorenzo.tarsitani@uniroma1.it

© Springer Nature Switzerland AG 2021
M. Biondi et al. (eds.), *Empathy, Normalization and De-escalation*,
https://doi.org/10.1007/978-3-030-65106-0_1

through clinical implications, we will try to disentangle this issue, providing a definition of agitation and aggression and framing both constructs in a theoretical and clinical perspective.

As Sacchetti et al. [3] note, currently there is not an unanimously shared definition of psychomotor agitation yet. The authors describe it as a "pathological condition characterized by a significant increase in ideation, emotional, motor and/or behavioral activity that may be associated with a variety of psychiatric and medical illnesses." Also, consistently with our dimensional conceptualization, Sacchetti et al. [3] note that clinical manifestations of agitation "go along a continuum ranging from a mere increase in ideation and behavioral activity to really acute and violent episodes." Similarly Lindenmayer [4] states "Motor restlessness, a heightened responsivity to external or internal stimuli, irritability, and inappropriate and usually purposeless verbal or motor activity are the hallmarks of the syndrome," including also decreased sleep and a significant fluctuation of symptoms over time. Citrome [5] underscores the importance of excessive motor or verbal activity, whether the fifth edition of the *Diagnostic and Statistical Manual of Mental Disorders* (DSM-5) [6] provides a more parsimonious definition "excessive motor activity associated with a feeling of inner tension. The activity is usually nonproductive and repetitious [...]." The Expert Consensus Panel for Behavioral Emergencies [7] describes the patient with psychomotor agitation as physically aggressive. Though agitation and aggression are frequently associated, aggression is not a core feature of psychomotor agitation [3], consistently with our theoretical approach. This is supported as well by the classification of subtypes of agitation [4] that identifies four distinct components: aggressive physical component; aggressive verbal component; non-aggressive physical component; and non-aggressive verbal component. Also, in some clinical conditions, e.g., acute anxiety conditions, patients might show agitation, but they are unlikely to be aggressive, with anxiety being a protective factor for risk of aggression (see Sect. 1.3).

It is also worth noting that the hallmarks of psychomotor agitation closely recall the core features of activation, which supports our conceptualization of agitation as a possible clinical expression of this psychopathological dimension. For instance, Pasquini and Bersani [8] state that "the concept of activation (or psychomotor activation) summarizes the psychopathological symptoms related to increased motor activity, agitation, acceleration of ideas, disinhibition, increased energy and self-confidence, euphoria, or irritability. Psychomotor activation is a disturbance of movement, cognition, and behaviour associated with psychiatric or physical conditions."

Though the term aggression is commonly used in a pejorative acceptation, it is actually a complex and multifaceted construct that needs to be clarified. Indeed, aggression does not necessarily fall within the field of psychopathology, as it represents an instinctual behavior with adaptive properties. The famous ethologist Konrad Lorenz in his book *On Aggression* [9] defines it as "the fighting instinct in beast and man which is directed against members of the same species." In an evolutionary psychological perspective, Buss and Duntley [10] hypothesize that aggression has some different functions: defending against attack, ascending dominance hierarchies, and promoting mating and reproduction (e.g., inflicting costs on sexual rivals). Aggression can be defined as an "overt action intended to harm" [11] or, more in detail, as "behavior directed by one individual against another individual (or object or self) with the aim of causing harm" [12]. Literature suggests that aggression is not a unitary phenomenon and it can be classified into subtypes. A major and long-standing distinction is between impulsive and instrumental aggression. The latter, also known as predatory aggression, is premeditated, goal-oriented, and usually initiated by the offender. It does not involve high levels of affect, but it is rather associated with callousness, whether the former arises abruptly as response to a perceived threat or provocation and involves an affective arousal with rage, anger, or hostility [13, 14]. Impulsive aggression is aimed at removing the obstacle to goal leading to frustration, which is a relevant trigger, as theorized by Dollard et al. [15]. It is worth recalling that, although a form of aggression can be predominant, both types of aggression can be observed in the same person, e.g., with antisocial personality disorder [16].

Another distinction that was validated both in children and adults is between reactive and proactive aggression. Such system resembles the previous classification, but these forms are not mutually exclusive, rather they are sub-dimensions contributing to one's general level of aggression [14]. Similarly, to the impulsive and predatory subtypes, respectively, reactive aggression is characterized by impulsivity and negative affect, whereas proactive aggression often involves psychopathic and callous traits.

Compared to predatory aggression, the impulsivity subtype is more commonly observed in psychiatric and medical settings, it is frequently associated with a range of clinical conditions (see Sect. 1.3), and it can be treated with pharmacological and non-pharmacological interventions. For such reason and for the clinical purpose of the current chapter, we will focus on impulsive aggression.

1.2 Epidemiology

Agitation is a common condition among psychiatric patients. In a literature overview, Sacchetti et al. [3] report in psychiatric emergency services a prevalence of agitation ranging from 4.3% to 10% [17–21]. Agitation is very common in schizophrenia, bipolar disorder's manic episode and mixed states, and dementia. Sacchetti et al. [22] reported that the prevalence of moderate or severe agitation in hospitalized patients with schizophrenia was 64.2%. The prevalence of agitation ranges between 19.5% and 87.9% [23–25] in patients with bipolar disorder and between 10% and 90% in patients with dementia [26]; whether 1.5% of all hospitalized patients [27] and 2.6% of patients in emergency room [28] were reported to show agitation.

Whether agitation is mainly to be considered a clinical manifestation, for the reasons we already addressed, aggression is a cross phenomenon that can be observed both in clinical and non-clinical individuals, and patients with untreated mental disorder (psychotic and mood disorders), substance use disorders, and both in comorbidity are more likely to be violent and aggressive than the general population. With no need of getting into deep with such issue, though, given the purpose of the current book, we will focus only on aggression in clinical populations. Scientific literature reports a prevalence of aggression ranging between 4.4% and 15% in psychiatric inpatients [17, 29–31]. The prevalence of use of restraint, which can be adopted as last intervention with overtly aggressive patients and can be considered as an indirect index of aggression in psychiatric wards, seems to support these data and falls between 7% and 12% according to many studies [32]. Schizophrenia is commonly associated with aggression, and hospitalized patients with schizophrenia show a prevalence of aggression ranging between 14% and 53.2% [31, 33], whether it is 8% in schizophrenic outpatients, but prevalence significantly increases up to 30% in individuals with substance abuse comorbidity [34]. Aggressive behaviors are also frequent among patients with first episode of psychosis (40% of patients presenting to services) [35], bipolar disorder (15% of discharged patients) [36], and dementia, with 22% [37] of the patients with mild/severe cognitive impairment in long-term facilities and 15.8% [38] of community patients with Alzheimer's disease presenting aggressive behaviors.

1.3   Clinical Conditions of Agitation and Aggression

As transdiagnostic dimensions, agitation and aggression can be observed in a wide range of conditions (Table 1.1). Many of them are primary psychiatric conditions, but they can be related to non-psychiatric, such neurological and medical conditions, and substance-related conditions. In most of the cases, agitation may co-occur in the same clinical picture. Most common primary psychiatric and neurodevelopmental disorders where both agitation and aggression can be observed are schizophrenia and other psychotic disorders, mania, borderline personality disorder, post-traumatic stress disorder and other trauma- and stressor-related disorders, dementia, intellectual disability, autism spectrum disorder, and attention deficit hyperactivity disorder. As well, agitation and aggression may be induced by both use and withdrawal of several substances such as alcohol, cocaine, amphetamines, steroids, ecstasy, phencyclidine, and others. Such substances represent potential causes per se, but they are also acknowledged to increase the risk of agitation and aggression in individuals with psychiatric disorders.

Among neuropsychiatric conditions, agitation and aggression are also commonly observed in dementia and virtually in any kind of confusional state (also called delirium). Common reasons of confusional state are medical internal conditions, e.g., systemic infection, HIV, hypoxia, electrolyte imbalance, excessive dose of medication, and neurological conditions, e.g., central nervous system infection (encephalitis, meningitis), head trauma, metabolic encephalopathy, and epilepsy.

It is worth noting that aggression and agitation can be observed in non-clinical conditions as well. Primary emotions such as anger, fear, and even happiness can induce different degrees of activation; anger generates aggressive behaviors as well

Table 1.1 Clinical and non-clinical conditions involving agitation, aggression, or both

Agitation	Both agitation and aggression	Aggression
Psychiatric, psychopathological, and psychological conditions		
	Schizophrenia and psychotic disorders	
	Mania	
Agitated depression		
Anxiety disorder (acute anxiety, panic attack)		
	Post-traumatic stress disorder and other trauma- and stressor-related disorders	
	Borderline personality disorder and other personality disorders	
		Antisocial personality disorder
		Paraphilias
		Intermittent explosive disorder and other disruptive, impulse control, and conduct disorders
	Emotional response (fear, anger) to acute stressors in non-clinical individuals	
Neurodevelopmental disorders		
	Intellectual disability	
	Autism spectrum disorder	
	Attention deficit hyperactivity disorder	
Substance use/intoxication/withdrawal		
	Alcohol	
	Cocaine and amphetamines	
	Ecstasy	
	Phencyclidine	
	Steroids	
	Other substances	
Neurocognitive disorders		
	Dementia	
	Delirium/confusional state	

as fear, activating the fight or flight response. According to this, aggression and agitation may be observed in non-clinical settings as consequence of an intense emotional response to acute or prolonged stressors.

With agitation and aggression being potentially observed together in a wide range of conditions and disorders, there are also some cases where they are unlikely to be associated. Acute anxiety conditions generate activation and agitation, but usually they are unlikely to result in aggressive behaviors. Similarly, patients with depression can manifest agitation (agitated depression), but aggression is uncommon.

Indeed, anxiety and depression are internalizing dimensions with inner focus, and actually they can be considered protective factors for aggression. In a previous study we conducted [32], negative affect, which include both anxiety and depression, was reported to reduce the risk of restraint, which can be considered an indirect measure of aggression in psychiatric intensive care units. Conversely, some other disorders include aggression among their typical symptoms, not necessarily being associated to agitation or where agitation plays a marginal role. Such disorders include all conditions where patients are more likely to display a form of cold aggression, which is typically planned and premeditated with a predatory goal. This can be observed, for instance, in paraphilic disorders such as pedophilia [39] and sexual sadism disorder. Also, individuals with antisocial personality disorder are likely to display cold aggression, though they can display impulsive aggression as well, where an emotional response is involved by definition and thus some degree of activation and even agitation can be possibly observed. Azevedo et al. [16] reported psychopathic traits to be a risk factor of premeditated aggression among patients with antisocial personality disorder. Finally, intermittent explosive disorder as well as other disruptive, impulse control, and conduct disorders includes aggression among their hallmarks. DSM-5 recognizes for such condition significant problems in both emotional and behavioral regulation, with more emphasis on one or the other aspect according to the specific disorder. For example, diagnostic criteria for the intermittent explosive disorder require aggression to be based on impulsive and/or anger and not premeditated and goal-oriented, which reasonably involve some degree of activation and agitation, as we already mentioned above for the antisocial personality disorder. Conversely this is not a criterion for conduct disorders where it is possible to specify if psychopathic traits are present, allowing both impulsive and cold aggression. Globally, although activation and agitation may occur together with aggression, they are not a typical manifestation of such disorders that rather include aggression as hallmark.

1.4   Neurobiology

As Rosell and Siever [14] noted in their interesting overview on aggression and violence, scientific studies on neurobiology focused their attention on the encephalic regions involved in impulse control, affect processing, and emotional decision-making. The amygdala, the orbitofrontal cortex and the anterior cingulate cortex, which belong to the limbic system, and the striatum (a nucleus in the subcortical basal ganglia) were reported to be involved in the neurobiology of aggression.

The amygdala is involved in emotional processing, and according to Rosell and Siever [14], reduced amygdala volumes, more labile activity, and higher responsivity to social threatening stimuli are associated with aggression. The orbitofrontal cortex and anterior cingulate cortex, which are interconnected with the amygdala, are involved in decision-making, emotional regulation, and reward-based learning, integrating affective and cognitive processes. Rosell and Siever [14] reported that aggression might be associated to decreased functional connectivity between the limbic, prefrontal cortex, and amygdala. Finally, the striatum and specifically its ventral portion are involved in determining the expected outcome value, e.g., expectations from social interaction. The authors hypothesize that dysfunction of the striatum might contribute to excessive frustration and therefore to subsequent higher risk of aggression.

In the context of neurotransmitters, literature addresses serotonin as the main neurotransmitter involved in the pathophysiology of aggression, even though dopamine, vasopressin, steroid hormones, and testosterone seem to play a role as well. For example, serotoninergic hypofunction [40], increased $5HT_{2A}$ receptor concentration and function in OFC, and reduced $5HT_{1A}$ binding potential in different areas were suggested to contribute to aggression and to explain its higher prevalence in males [14, 41, 42].

Because of its complexity and the number of possible underlying causes, the neuroanatomy and biology of agitation are not well understood yet. Sachdev and Kruk [43] proposed a neurobiological model for restlessness, which is a core feature of agitation, involving the striatum, pallidum, thalamus, and cortex, with the striatum and prefrontal cortex playing a main role. According to the authors, restlessness might be due to disturbances of such circuits that, depending on the etiopathogenesis of the underlying condition, can be caused by a number of different pathophysiological mechanisms [4]. They include increase in dopamine in psychosis, mania, and substance-induced agitation and decrease in GABA in dementia, anxiety, where increase in norepinephrine is involved as well, and agitated depression, where decrease in GABA is associated to increased serotoninergic responsivity. In confusional states, mechanisms are not univocal because of the different underlying conditions. Finally, according to Lyndenmayer [4], an increased noradrenergic and decreased serotoninergic activity may represent the underlying mechanism in conditions associated with agitation.

It is worth noting that the proposed pathophysiological models share some nodal common regions such as the striatum and the orbitofrontal cortex. This partial neurobiological overlapping might contribute to explain the common co-occurrence of agitation and aggression in several conditions.

1.5 Agitation and Aggression: Settings and Clinical Implications

Both agitation and aggression, especially if acute or if they reach severe degrees, may represent emergency conditions, requiring a prompt intervention that can drastically change its evolution [44]. It is worth recalling that in the following paragraphs, we will consider only the impulsive aggression subtype which is more likely to be observed in psychiatric and medical settings and to be associated to psychopathological conditions.

As potential emergency conditions, agitation and aggression can be easily observed in psychiatric emergency services and psychiatric intensive care units (PICU). In Italy, though different models are possible, psychiatric emergency services are always hospital-based, and a key role is played by the emergency room (ER), where individuals with acute psychiatric conditions can present to, either voluntarily or compulsorily. Usually they follow a common pathway independently from the primary reason of complaint; they are assessed by an emergency physician and usually undergo blood and instrumental exams. Emergency physicians might ask for an urgent psychiatric evaluation provided by a consultant psychiatrist from the PICU who will decide whether or not prescribing a medication, suggesting further exams and, above all, admitting the patient to the PICU or refer him or her to a community service.

In the following paragraphs, we will discuss our experience in both emergency setting and PICU, reporting the results of two studies we conducted in a dimensional perspective.

1.5.1   Agitation and Aggression in Psychiatric Emergency Service: Introduction and Methods

The current paragraph focuses on the findings of our research group from a study that we conducted. Here we summarized the main information on setting and participants; for details, see Dazzi et al. [45].

The study was conducted at the University Hospital Policlinico Umberto I in Rome, Italy, which is the largest university hospital in Italy; it serves a crowded metropolitan catchment area and receives a varied population, with one third of the patients coming from other regions or even other countries. We recruited 312 patients presenting to the ER for whom a psychiatric consultation was required. For all patients, we collected sociodemographic and clinical data, and a dimensional evaluation was performed by a senior psychiatrist using the SVARAD, a dimensional assessment tool that includes ten psychopathological dimensions: apprehension/fear, sadness/demoralization, anger/aggressiveness, obsessiveness, apathy, impulsivity, reality distortion, thought disorganization, somatic preoccupation/somatization, and activation. Each dimension can be rated on a 5-points scale, ranging from absent to profound [2].

For the current chapter, additional analyses were performed. Student's t-test or ANOVA with Bonferroni post hoc tests was used to compare quantitative data among different groups. SVARAD dimensions were considered as quantitative variables. Chi-square was used to compare qualitative data, e.g., categorical diagnosis, main reason of assessment, proposal for compulsory admission, and recommended admission. After a statistically significant chi-square test, standardized residuals (SR) were considered as a post hoc test for cell significance. Observed values were considered to significantly differ from the expected value when the standardized residuals (SR) had a value greater than 2.0 (>2.0 or <−2.0). To analyze the correlation between the SVARAD dimensions, we performed the Pearson correlation analysis. Finally, we performed a two-step cluster analysis of the SVARAD dimensions and assigned patients to one of the clusters.

As usual, the level of significance was set at 0.05.

In the current paragraph, after presenting descriptive data, we will first analyze the primary reason for consultation, focusing on psychomotor agitation and impulse/behavioral dyscontrol and its clinical implications. Then, consistently with a dimensional approach, as we mentioned in the Introduction of this chapter, we will focus on the psychopathological dimensions underlying agitation and aggression, i.e., activation and aggressiveness, with some consideration to impulsivity as well that can be associated both to agitation and aggression. We will go through the association between these dimensions and other clinical data and discuss the implication. Finally, we will focus on the dimensional clusters and their implications.

1.5.2   Primary Reason of Psychiatric in Emergency Room

The mean age of the sample was 40.1 years, and the gender distribution was balanced; almost one fifth of the sample was foreign; the diagnostic areas were distributed as follows: psychotic disorders 24.5%, bipolar disorders 12.6%, depressive disorders 18.2%, anxiety disorders 13.2%, and other diagnoses 31.5%. About one patient out of eight reached the ER with a proposal for compulsory admission[1].

Psychiatric consultation was required for a number of reasons; psychomotor agitation was the most frequent (21.5%), whereas impulse/behavioral dyscontrol, which includes aggression, accounted for 10.9%. The distribution of the reasons for psychiatric consultation is displayed in Table 1.2.

As we could expect, consistently with our initial hypothesis, patients with psychomotor agitation and impulse/behavioral dyscontrol showed significantly higher degrees of activation ($p < 0.001$), anger/aggressiveness ($p < 0.001$), and impulsivity ($p < 0.001$), compared to most of the other reasons for consultation. The highest mean level of activation was observed in patients with psychomotor agitation, whereas anger/aggressiveness reached the highest mean level in patients with

Table 1.2 Primary reasons for psychiatric consultation

Reason for consultation	n	%
Confusional state	19	6.3
Delusional/hallucinatory state	51	16.9
PMA	65	21.5
Depressive state	35	11.6
Self-harming	45	14.9
IBD	33	10.9
Anxiety	25	8.3
Other	29	9.6

Numbers may not add up due to missing data
Percentages refer to valid cases
PMA psychomotor agitation, *IBD* impulse/behavioral dyscontrol

[1] According to Italian law, the procedure for compulsory admission requires two physicians to be involved: the first one signs the proposal, and the second one, usually a psychiatrist, decides whether to confirm it or not.

psychomotor agitation. More in detail, using Bonferroni post hoc tests, we did not observe any statistical difference in mean activation, anger/aggressiveness, and impulsivity between patients with psychomotor agitation or impulse/behavioral dyscontrol. As well, no differences were observed for the other SVARAD dimensions except for apprehension/fear that was significantly higher in patients with psychomotor agitation (1.8 ± 1 vs. 1.1 ± 1). Conversely, patients with psychomotor agitation showed significantly higher levels of activation than all the other groups except for delusional/hallucinatory states; the same difference was observed for those with impulse/behavioral dyscontrol, although activation was not significantly higher compared to groups with delusional/hallucinatory states and self-harming behavior. Similarly, mean level of anger/aggressiveness was significantly higher than all the other groups except for self-harm behavior. Finally, impulsivity reached its highest level in patients with self-harm behavior, where it was significantly higher than all the other groups. Impulsivity was also higher in patients with psychomotor agitation and impulse/behavioral dyscontrol only compared to depressive and anxiety states and other.

The mean levels of activation, anger/aggressiveness, and impulsivity across main reasons why psychiatric assessment was required are displayed in Fig. 1.1.

Psychomotor agitation was significantly more likely ($p < 0.001$) to be observed in patients with bipolar disorder (BPD; 18 out of 35), whereas it is worth noting that more than half of the patients (17 out of 32) displaying impulse/behavioral dyscontrol did not fall within any of the major diagnostic areas (psychotic, depression, bipolar, and anxiety disorders), and rather they were significantly much more likely

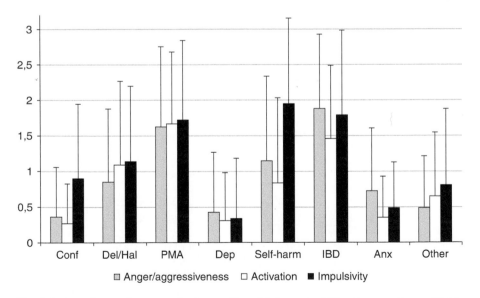

Fig. 1.1 Anger/aggressiveness, activation, and impulsivity across different reasons for psychiatric assessment. *Conf* confusional state, *Del/Hal* delusional/hallucinatory state, *PMA* psychomotor agitation, *Dep* depressive state, *Self-harm* self-harming behavior, *IBD* impulse/behavioral dyscontrol, *Anx* anxiety state

to be diagnosed as "Other," which included half cases (8/17) of substance abuse/ intoxication. Psychotic disorders were not associated to impulse/behavioral dyscontrol or psychomotor agitation as main reason of complaint; rather delusional/hallucinatory states were the most frequent main reason of assessment. Since psychomotor agitation can be frequently observed in psychosis, this finding might be counterintuitive, but it is worth recalling that we evaluated only the primary reason of assessment as a mutually exclusive variable; thus a delusional/hallucinatory state does not exclude a certain degree of psychomotor agitation; rather it means that the delusional/hallucinatory state was considered as more relevant by the physician requiring the psychiatric consultation. On the other hand, the comparison of SVARAD psychopathological dimensions among diagnostic groups pointed that only Reality Distortion and Thought Disorganization were systematically higher in psychosis compared to the other diagnostic groups (except for BPD where Thought Disorganization was only slightly but not significantly lower), whereas activation ($p < 0.001$), anger/aggressiveness ($p < 0.001$), and impulsivity ($p < 0.001$) were not significantly higher in almost every comparison, rather lower when compared to BPD. This finding is consistent with the heterogeneity of schizophrenia and schizophrenic spectrum disorders, where activation is just one facet of a complex dimensional picture that includes positive symptoms, negative symptoms, disorganization, activation, and depression, with different dimensions prevailing from patient to patient [46].

Unlike those with psychomotor agitation, patients with IBD as main reason of assessment were also more likely to reach the ER with a proposal for compulsory admission ($p < 0.001$), but both groups were not significantly more likely to be recommended for psychiatric admission (the rate of recommended admission for psychomotor agitation was 36.9%, for impulse/behavioral dyscontrol was 42.4%, for the total sample was 39.4%). Patients with psychomotor agitation were significantly more likely to be treated in ER ($p < 0.001$) either with benzodiazepines, antipsychotics, or a combination of them, whereas those with impulse/behavioral dyscontrol were not.

1.5.3 Dimensional Approach to Agitation and Aggression and Psychopathological Clusters in ER

Consistently with our theoretical model, we also focused on the clinical implications of the psychopathological dimensions underlying agitation and aggression, i.e., activation, anger/aggressiveness, and impulsivity.

Patients who reached the ER with a proposal of compulsory admission showed significantly higher levels of activation, anger/aggressiveness, and impulsivity, as well as those for who were recommended to be admitted, even though as we reported in a previous paper [45] only impulsivity was an independent predictor for recommended admission.

Patients who were treated with antipsychotics, alone or in association with benzodiazepines, showed significantly higher activation, anger/aggressiveness, and

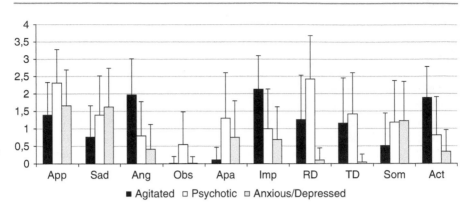

Fig. 1.2 SVARAD dimensions for each psychopathological cluster. Data are displayed as mean ± standard deviation. *App* apprehension/fear, *Sad* sadness/demoralization, *Ang* anger/aggressiveness, *Obs* obsessiveness, *Apa* apathy, *Imp* impulsivity, *RD* reality distortion, *TD* thought disorganization, *Som* somatic preoccupation/somatization, *ACT* activation

impulsivity, whether those who were treated with benzodiazepines alone showed higher activation, but no significant difference was observed for anger/aggressiveness and impulsivity. No significant difference in between gender was observed.

Activation, anger/aggressiveness, and impulsivity show a significant correlation ($p < 0.01$ with Pearson correlation coefficient ranging between 0.52 and 0.63); they can be clustered together and framed as outer dimensions [8]. We performed a two-step cluster analysis including all the SVARAD dimensions that pointed three different psychopathological clusters, labeled as agitated ($n = 107$), psychotic ($n = 69$), and anxious/depressed ($n = 136$) cluster. The agitated cluster was characterized by striking symptoms with relevant degrees of activation, anger/aggressiveness, and impulsivity. The psychopathological profile of each cluster is displayed in Fig. 1.2.

Patients assigned to the agitated cluster, which represent over one third of the overall sample, were significantly more likely to reach the ER with a proposal of compulsory admission, accounting for 71% of the total, to be assessed for psychomotor agitation (40.0%), impulse/behavioral dyscontrol (21.0%), or self-harm behavior (17.1%) as primary reason, to be treated with antipsychotics alone or in association with benzodiazepines, and to be diagnosed with BPD. The rate of recommended admission (48.6% vs. 39.6% in the whole sample) was not significantly higher in this group. Also, the rate of compulsory admission in this group was high (10 out of 17 patients), but the difference we observed was not statistically significant presumably due to the small number of compulsorily admitted sample.

Both in the total sample and in the agitated cluster patients who reached the ER with a proposal for compulsory admission were much more likely to be compulsorily hospitalized (43.6% and 35.7%, respectively; $p < 0.001$). Though this finding seems intuitive, it deserves to be more deeply discussed. Indeed, in a relevant part of the sample, the compulsory proposal was not confirmed. A few cases were not even admitted whether 42.9% of the patients could be admitted to PICU voluntarily. Data are displayed in Table 1.3. According to our experience, compulsory admission might be proposed inappropriately in a small number of patients, where

Table 1.3 Compulsory admission, voluntary admission, and discharge distribution across patients reaching the ER with or without proposal of compulsory admission, both in the total sample and in the agitated cluster

	Compulsory admission N (%)	Voluntary admission N (%)	Discharge N (%)
Agitated cluster			
Proposed for CA	10 (35.7)	12 (42.9)	6 (21.4)
Not proposed for CA	0 (0)	29 (37.2)	49 (62.8)
Total sample			
Proposed for CA	17 (43.6)	14 (35.9)	8 (20.5)
Not proposed for CA	0 (0)	86 (32.0)	180 (68.0)

Numbers may not add up due to missing data
Percentages refer to valid cases
CA compulsory admission

inappropriate clinical pictures are present (e.g., substance intoxication) or social conditions prevail. This explanation might presumably account for part of the patients that were actually discharged. More notably in a clinically significant number of patients, consent to admission could be recovered and compulsory admission be avoided, both in the total and agitated sample. Though this observation is based on a small number of cases and further research is deserved, it might show interesting implication, not limited to agitated patients, for the application of the END method in acute psychiatric settings.

1.5.4 Overall Considerations

Agitation and aggression are frequent conditions, and together they account for almost one third of all the reasons for psychiatric consultation. The results support our initial hypothesis that activation and anger/aggressiveness are the psychopathological core dimensions underlying agitation and aggression, respectively, with impulsivity being involved as well but playing a less specific role. As literature suggests, they are more frequent in some specific conditions, but they can be detected in almost every clinical picture which qualifies them as transdiagnostic.

Agitation and aggression frequently co-occur, they are likely to be observed together in the same clinical condition, and the underlying dimensions are strongly inter-correlated as well. Although some differences can be observed, our results failed to clearly discriminate the psychopathological profiles between psychomotor agitation and impulse/behavioral dyscontrol that were rather quite similar. However, about only a half of the patients with high degrees (severe or profound) of activation showed high degrees of anger/aggressiveness as well and vice versa which means that in about half of the cases, patients are likely to show a clinical picture with either activation or anger/aggressiveness prevailing. Overall, such findings yield a twofold consideration: on one hand, as literature suggests, agitation and aggression, as well as their core underlying dimensions, seem to be at least partially independent, and they can be observed separately; on the other hand though, in a clinical perspective, the frequent co-occurrence of agitation and aggression and the strong correlation between the underlying dimensions, impulsivity included, suggest that patients showing clinical signs of any of these dimensions might have a greater risk of presenting symptoms or behavior that typically belongs to the other psychopathological dimensions. For example, patients with agitation might be more easily become aggressive and impulsive. While complex clinical conditions involving agitation, aggression, and impulsivity often require both pharmacological and non-pharmacological intervention, aimed to comprehensively treat the whole clinical picture, we hypothesize that patients showing only one of these dimensions prevailing might still benefit from a non-pharmacological preventive intervention targeted at reducing the symptoms of all the outer dimensions, in order to avoid a potential escalation.

Patients assessed for psychomotor agitation and impulse/behavioral dyscontrol and generally those who were assigned to the agitated cluster did not show a significantly higher rate of recommended admission. This finding might be apparently unexpected, but it can be presumably explained according to the heterogeneous reasons of agitation and aggression. Indeed, agitation and aggression can be due to a number of causes, but only some of them should be considered properly as psychopathological and psychiatric conditions. For example, acute confusional states are better managed in different settings, according to the underlying cause; patients with either acute intoxication or dementia showing aggression and agitation might require an acute intervention in ER, but they might not benefit from a longer hospitalization in PICU if no other major psychiatric disorders are associated. Finally, in a non-negligible part of the cases, emergency psychiatry is still improperly claimed to play a custodial role to face non-clinical conditions where social problems actually prevail.

Finally, though the proposal for compulsory admission is a strong predictor of effective compulsory admission, as expected, it is worth underscoring that in a relevant number of cases, an adequate intervention in ER can help retrieving therapeutic alliance and consent to hospitalization, avoiding compulsorily admission and its well-known negative psychological consequences. Though further specific research is deserved to better clarify this issue, according to our experience, we believe that non-pharmacological intervention might play a key role to this aim.

1.6   Agitation and Aggression in Psychiatric Intensive Care Unit

Psychomotor agitation and aggression are significant risks and challenges in psychiatric intensive care units, with particular emphasis just after admission and during the first days after. Nurse and medical staff work several times with these patients under a heavy pressure, both diligence and fear. They often work under the risk of attacks and of physical injuries. Sometimes they suffer because of these issues, both at emotional and physical levels, with the risk of physical injuries. Safety rules of the organization and of the structure of the ward, working in team and, particularly, being trained in communication with patients, are needed. Dealing with such kind of risk is, in any way, a complex task giving the complexity and multifactor aspects of agitation, aggression, and violence, as well as the unpredictability of the reactions of some patients.

From a clinical viewpoint, psychomotor agitation and anger bursts along with aggressiveness are commonly reported in psychiatric patients with acute psychopathology, particularly in patients with psychotic disorders or with substance use and related disorders.

As aforementioned (see Sect. 1.3), psychomotor agitation and aggression are more frequent in a number of clinical conditions, even though we observed in a previous study [1] that they can be detected in the whole psychiatric population, of course at a lesser extent than psychotic and substance use disorders [1]. However, the categorical diagnostic approach by means of DSM-5 or the tenth edition of the *International Classification of Diseases* (ICD-10) is not useful as expected, because of the wide variance of clinical pictures of such disorders in their acute phase. A clinical approach according to prevalent psychopathological "dimensions" is more useful than a categorical approach in describing and predicting aggressive and violent behaviors. Psychopathological dimensions' profiles usefully describe the predominant components of suffering, regardless of the categorical diagnosis [1].

In emergency psychiatry, high levels of activation and psychomotor agitation, as well aggressiveness, are a frequent reason for admission independently from the categorical diagnosis. They also often represent a difficult issue for treatment adherence to treatment, relationship with the staff, community activities, and therapeutic alliance.

A dimensional approach to diagnosis, together with ICD and DSM-IV (now DSM-5) categorical model, has been used for many years both in clinical practice and for research purpose at the Department of Neurosciences and Mental Health of Policlinico Umberto I University Hospital of Rome [2]. The dimensional assessment was made using SVARAD, which is routinely administered at admission and at discharge. The dimensional assessment guides the pharmacological and psychological treatment, as well as the approach and communication to the patients; clinicians and healthcare professionals use the dimensional profiles achieved from the dimensional assessment to frame the psychopathological suffering of a patient and to use the right technique to establish the best communication. In most cases, the right communication with the aggressive and agitated patient avoids the necessity of a compulsory treatment and allows voluntary hospitalization and a better climate to deal with the necessary treatment (psychosocial or pharmacological treatment).

We preliminarily describe here data from an observational study of 847 psychiatric inpatients, admitted to the acute ward at our hospital assessed with the SVARAD instrument. The sample of inpatients had 11.8 days of mean length of stay in psychiatric ward, and 16.3% had involuntary type of admission, with 16.5% attempted suicide requiring admission. All the patients received DSM-IV or ICD-10 categorical diagnosis by experienced clinicians with supervision of the senior chief psychiatrist. The psychopathological assessment was based on the SVARAD dimensions (see Sect. 1.5.1) The SVARAD profiles showed a very interesting variability of suffering within the same diagnostic DSM-IV or ICD-10 clinical group.

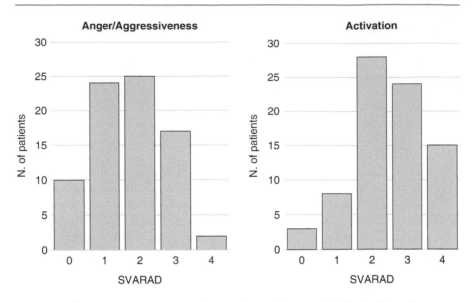

Figs. 1.3 and 1.4 SVARAD scores for the anger/aggressiveness and activation dimensions across inpatients with bipolar disorder, hypomanic/manic episode (*N* = 78). (Source: [1])

In our dimensional assessment, the dimension anger/aggressiveness is defined as "Feelings of irritation, resentment and anger; display of irritability, litigiousness, hostility; verbal or physical violence." The dimension activation is defined as "Increased motor activity; racing thoughts, disinhibition; feelings of excessive confidence; euphoria or irritability."

As concerns anger/aggressiveness, findings were exciting because this dimension was present not in just one or two diagnostic categories but in several ones. This knowledge guides the clinician to recognize needs of each patient, quite apart from the type of psychotic, personality, and affective diagnoses. It also guides to the communication skills to adopt, such as empathic communication, normalization, and, especially, de-escalation techniques. Higher levels of anger/aggressiveness resulted in bipolar disorder manic episode and then in decompensated borderline personality disorder, bipolar mixed episode, psychotic disorder NOS, schizoaffective disorder, and with schizophrenia as the sixth one. Of interest was the variance within a same diagnostic category. For instance, among the 31 patients with schizophrenia, 14 had no anger/aggressiveness rate at all, while 4 had mild, 6 moderate, and 5 severe.

Below we show some examples of our inpatient sample in which the anger/aggressiveness and activation dimensions stand out in particular.

In the bipolar sample with hypomanic/manic episode (*N* = 78), moderate values of the dimension anger/aggressiveness were found in 25 patients, mild in 24 patients, severe in 18 patients, profound in 3 patients, and absent in 10 patients, while moderate values of the dimension activation were found in 28 patients, mild in 8 patients, severe in 24 patients, and profound in 15 patients, and the dimension was absent in 3 patients (Figs. 1.3 and 1.4).

In the bipolar disorder mixed episode ($N = 34$), as concerns the dimension anger/aggressiveness, 12 patients were rated mild, 7 patients moderate, 7 patients severe, and 9 patients absent, while moderate values of the dimension activation were found in 13 patients, severe in 4 patients, and profound in 2 patients.

Case Vignette 1

A. is a patient with manic bipolar disorder and has been admitted for some days in the intensive psychiatry unit. Despite psychopharmacological therapy, he has so far shown only small improvements: he shows agitation as a result of its delusional themes of greatness and tries to leave the ward. When prevented, the patient shows aggressive behavior towards doctors and nurses.

The doctor approaches the patient and says in a very calm way: "Mr. A, I see that you are quite agitated, there must be something that really made you angry …"

The patient looks at him and in a loud voice replies: "Of course, I can't go out! I am no longer a free man! This is why I am really angry with you all assholes. Let me go, otherwise I will call the police."

The doctor now has two nurses next to him who are about 1 m away and says to him: "Of course, I guess it must be difficult for you to feel this way. I'm sorry because I understand that you are suffering (Empathic Communication)."

The patient replies: "I am suffering but nobody seems to understand it, nobody listens to me! You just want to prevent me from going out."

The doctor says calmly but respectfully: "Mr. A … listen? Of course we listen to you, explain to me. This is where I listen to you as long as you want."

The patient begins to explain why he has to go out, because of his delusional themes and why he has to do many things.

The doctor says to him: "Of course, I know he has to do many things and your mind runs, that he has many ideas. Sometimes it happens to some people to have periods like this, it has happened to others too. Sometimes, however, when there are many things to do, these have to be planned well otherwise you risk hurting them. It is normal for haste and urgency to lead to mistakes and it is normal for a person to feel stuck getting angry. I would like to talk to you about your plans and that explain better, let's talk (Normalization)."

The patient at this point shows himself less aggressive and begins to speak a little.

The doctor adds: "I realize that it is a complex situation, tell me how we can help it. Since I feel that you are very agitated and angry, I can give you some medication that help you calm down a little so you can speak better (De-escalation)."

The patient accepts drug therapy and the crisis situation resolves (Figs. 1.5, 1.6, 1.7, and 1.8).

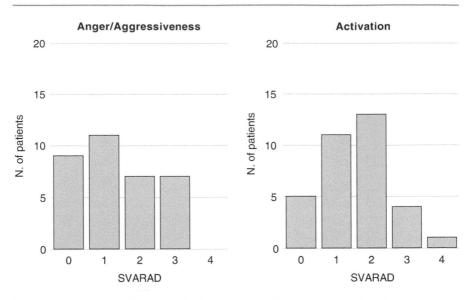

Figs. 1.5 and 1.6 SVARAD scores for the anger/aggressiveness and activation dimensions across inpatients with bipolar disorder, mixed episode ($N = 34$). (Source: [1])

As concerns activation, severe-profound levels were found mostly in the bipolar hypomanic/manic episode and the bipolar mixed episode, in schizoaffective and psychotic disorder NOS, and then in schizophrenia and borderline personality disorder.

In summary, anger/aggressiveness and activation/agitation SVARAD dimensions were present in all the diagnostic DSM-IV groups, peaking in hypomanic/manic episode, mixed bipolar episode decompensated borderline disorder, psychotic disorder NOS, and schizoaffective disorder. The very high peaking severe to profound of the activation dimension in the bipolar hypomanic/manic patients should be carefully considered. These findings suggest a major clinical target for approaching the patient according to the END technique. These psychopathological dimensions of suffering seem to be the more relevant target to be addressed in the therapeutic communication and patient-therapist relationship. The issue is also relevant concerning problems of safety for the nurse and medical staff in the prevention of aggressive and violent acting outs and behavior (Fig. 1.9).

High activation and anger/aggressiveness are severe obstacles for the communication with patient: they often arise from perception of imminent threat, persecutory ideation, and feeling of fear or terror; they are subsequent to the breakdown of psychic defense under psychotic disorganization, as well as the vicissitudes of emergency, with police or officers intervention, the ambulance team, and the need of a temporary compulsory intervention. The empathic communication is particularly useful in this phase (see below) to reach a relationship, accept the psychologist or psychiatrist, and, then, start with de-escalation and negotiating techniques. They are the basis for the building of a "good enough" therapeutic alliance, introducing drug

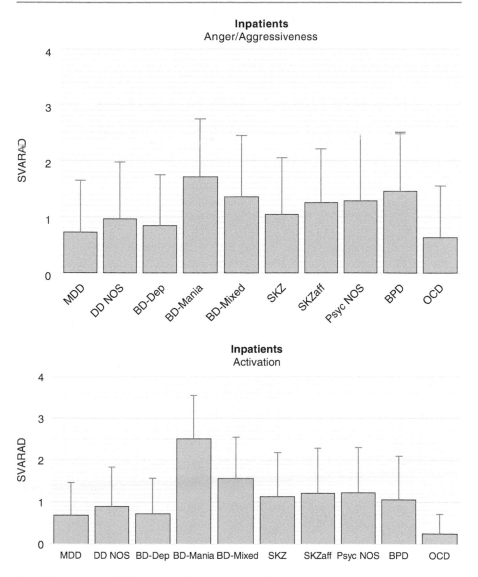

Figs. 1.7 and 1.8 SVARAD anger/aggressiveness (first figure) and activation (second figure) dimension across inpatients' diagnostic categories: mean values and standard deviations. *MDD* major depressive disorder; *DDNOS* depressive disorder not otherwise specified; *BP-Dep* bipolar disorder, depressive episode; *BP-Mania* bipolar disorder, manic episode; *BP-Mixed* bipolar disorder, mixed episode; *SKZ* schizophrenia; *SKZaff* schizoaffective disorder; *PsycNOS* psychotic disorder not otherwise specified; *BPD* borderline personality disorder; *OCD* obsessive compulsive disorder. (Source: [1])

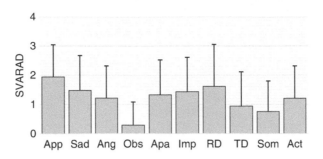

Fig. 1.9 SVARAD profile of the whole psychiatric sample ($N = 847$): mean scores and standard deviations of the inpatients group. *App* apprehension/fear, *Sad* sadness/demoralization, *Ang* anger/aggressiveness, *Obs* obsessiveness, *Apa* apathy, *Imp* impulsivity, *RD* reality distortion, *TD* thought disorganization, *Som* somatic preoccupation/somatization, *ACT* activation. (Source: [1])

treatment and explaining recent events leading to admission and acceptance of treatment and of a therapeutic project. In our experience, this approach of communication addressed to psychopathological dimension, rather than to the specific clinical diagnosis (i.e., schizophrenia rather than bipolar disorder), led to decrease of compulsory treatment and contention.

Courses for nurses and doctors are currently being held to teach END communication. This is part of a program established by the hospital, precisely to help healthcare professionals manage difficult situations with patients, not necessarily psychiatrists who experience agitation, but, for example, in preoperative or postoperative situations, and anger and aggression behavior, or even in the management of communication with relatives of hospitalized patients.

Case Vignette 2

Mrs. G. has her husband hospitalized in a surgery ward and wants to come in to find him outside the visiting hours while the nursing team is medicating and working on the patients. The lady rings the door several times and shouts. She seems very anxious and agitated. At that moment a ward doctor arrives and is returning from a consultation. The lady attacks him aloud and says in a very angry tone: "Let me in! I want to see how my husband is doing. If I don't think about him, you treat him badly! Don't let me in, I'm his wife!"

The doctor replies: "Madam, I guess you are very worried about your husband. I understand that you would like to be able to do more for him (Empathic Communication). It is normal to feel this way if your husband has been operated a few days ago (Normalization). You can come in later to see him; in the meantime can I help you? Is there anything you want to ask me? I assure you that as soon as I enter the ward, I go to greet him and tell him that you are out and waiting to see him (De-escalation)."

In this case, the use of the END method was rapid and sequential, achieving the aim of making the lady feel that the doctor understood her state of mind, offering a normalizing response and de-escalating action.

1.7   Conclusions

In conclusion, psychomotor agitation and aggression are frequently observed in medical, psychiatric, and non-clinical settings. They represent the behavioral expression of activation and aggressiveness, which are transdiagnostic psychopathological dimensions. They can be present in range medical conditions, especially in acute confusional states, and they can also represent a reaction in healthy individuals. Individuals with mental disorders, like psychotic and mood disorders, but also personality disorders are at higher risk of psychomotor agitation and aggression. Substance use and withdrawal are associated with agitation and aggression in persons with and without mental disorders.

Psychomotor agitation and aggression frequently co-occur, been agitation a possible predictor of aggressive and impulsive behavior.

Despite possible underlined clinical condition, even few signs of these dimensions benefit from a non-pharmacological preventive intervention to avoid potential escalation.

In psychiatric emergency settings, patients with psychomotor agitation and impulse/behavioral dyscontrol do not always show higher rates of admission in wards, due to the heterogeneity of the phenomenon.

Patients assessed in ER with proposal for compulsory psychiatric admission are frequently agitated, impulsive, and aggressive. However, adequate communication intervention in ER can be effective in retrieving therapeutic alliance and consent to hospitalization.

A dimensional approach to individuals with high levels of agitation and/or aggressiveness can be very useful in guiding communication interventions, such as empathic communication, normalization, and de-escalation techniques.

References

1. Biondi M, Pasquini M, Picardi A. Dimensional psychopathology. Berlin: Springer International Publishing; 2018.
2. Pancheri P, Biondi M, Gaetano P, Picardi A. Costruzione della "SVARAD" una scala per la valutazione rapida dimensionale. Riv Psichiatr. 1999;36:204–16.
3. Sacchetti E. Psychomotor agitation in psychiatry: an Italian expert consensus. Evid Bas Psychiatr Care. 2017;3:1–24.
4. Lindenmayer JP. The pathophysiology of agitation. J Clin Psychiatry. 2000;61:5–10.
5. Citrome L. Addressing the need for rapid treatment of agitation in schizophrenia and bipolar disorder: focus on inhaled loxapine as an alternative to injectable agents. Ther Clin Risk Manag. 2013;9:235–45.
6. American Psychiatric Association. Diagnostic and statistical manual of mental disorders. 5th ed. Arlington, VA: American Psychiatric Publishing; 2013.
7. Allen MH, Currier GW, Hughes DH, Docherty JP, Carpenter D, Ross R. Treatment of behavioral emergencies: a summary of the expert consensus guidelines. J Psychiatr Pract. 2003;9:16–38.
8. Bersani FS, Pasquini M. The "outer dimensions": impulsivity, anger/aggressiveness, activation. In: Biondi M, Pasquini M, Picardi A, editors. Dimensional psychopathology. Berlin: Springer International Publishing; 2018.

9. Lorenz K. On aggression. London: Methuen; 1966.
10. Buss DM, Duntley JD. The evolution of aggression. In: Schaller M, Simpson J, Kenrick DT, editors. Evolution and social psychology. New York, NY: Psychology Press; 2013. p. 263–86.
11. Volavka J. Violence in schizophrenia and bipolar disorder. Psychiatr Danub. 2013;25:24–33.
12. Bond AJ. Pharmacological manipulation of aggressiveness and impulsiveness in healthy volunteers. Prog Neuropsychopharmacol Biol Psychiatry. 1992;16:1–7.
13. Penders T, Freudenreich O, Leentjens AFG, Soellner W, Peterson T, Rummans T, et al. Aggression and violence an evidence-based medicine (EBM) monograph for psychosomatic medicine practice: Academy of Psychosomatic Medicine (APM) and the European Association of Psychosomatic Medicine (EAPM); 2013. p. 1–22.
14. Rosell DR, Siever LJ. The neurobiology of aggression and violence. CNS Spectr. 2015;20:254–79.
15. Boring EG, Dollard J, Doob LW, Miller NE, Mowrer OH, Sears RR, et al. Frustration and aggression. Am J Psychol. 1939;52:480–3.
16. Azevedo J, Vieira-Coelho M, Castelo-Branco M, Coelho R, Figueiredo-Braga M. Impulsive and premeditated aggression in male offenders with antisocial personality disorder. PLoS One. 2020;15:e0229876.
17. Tardiff K, Sweillam A. Assaultive behavior among chronic inpatients. Am J Psychiatry. 1982;139:212–5.
18. Oliva-Moreno J, López-Bastida J, Osuna-Guerrero R, Montejo-González AL, Duque-González B. The costs of schizophrenia in spain. Eur J Health Econ. 2006;7:179–84.
19. Pascual JC, Madre M, Puigdemont D, Oller S, Corripio I, Díaz A, et al. A naturalistic study: 100 consecutive episodes of acute agitation in a psychiatric emergency department. Actas Esp Psiquiatr. 2006;34:239–44.
20. Sachs GS. A review of agitation in mental illness: burden of illness and underlying pathology. J Clin Psychiatry. 2006;67:5–12.
21. Huf G, Alexander J, Gandhi P, Allen MH. Haloperidol plus promethazine for psychosis-induced aggression. Cochrane Database Syst Rev. 2016;11:CD005146.
22. Sacchetti E, Valsecchi P, Tamussi E, Paulli L, Morigi R, Vita A. Psychomotor agitation in subjects hospitalized for an acute exacerbation of Schizophrenia. Psychiatry Res. 2018;270:357–64.
23. Spitzer RL, Endicott J, Robins E. Research diagnostic criteria: rationale and reliability. Arch Gen Psychiatry. 1978;35:773–82.
24. Maj M, Pirozzi R, Magliano L, Bartoli L. Agitated depression in bipolar I disorder: prevalence, phenomenology, and outcome. Am J Psychiatry. 2003;160:2134–40.
25. Serretti A, Olgiati P. Profiles of "manic" symptoms in bipolar I, bipolar II and major depressive disorders. J Affect Disord. 2005;84:159–66.
26. Bartels SJ, Horn SD, Smout RJ, Dums AR, Flaherty E, Jones JK, et al. Agitation and depression in frail nursing home elderly patients with dementia: treatment characteristics and service use. Am J Geriatr Psychiatry. 2003;11:231–8.
27. Cots F, Chiarello P, Pérez V, Gracia A, Becerra V. Hospital costs associated with agitation in the acute care setting. Psychiatr Serv. 2016;67:124–7.
28. Miner JR, Klein LR, Cole JB, Driver BE, Moore JC, Ho JD. The characteristics and prevalence of agitation in an urban county emergency department. Ann Emerg Med. 2018;72:361–70.
29. Grassi L, Biancosino B, Marmai L, Kotrotsiou V, Zanchi P, Peron L, et al. Violence in psychiatric units: a 7-year Italian study of persistently assaultive patients. Soc Psychiatry Psychiatr Epidemiol. 2006;41:698–703.
30. Biancosino B, Delmonte S, Grassi L, Santone G, Preti A, Miglio R, et al. Violent behavior in acute psychiatric inpatient facilities: a national survey in italy. J Nerv Ment Dis. 2009;197:772–82.
31. Zhou JS, Zhong BL, Xiang YT, Chen Q, Cao XL, Correll CU, et al. Prevalence of aggression in hospitalized patients with schizophrenia in China: a meta-analysis. Asia Pac Psychiatry. 2016;8:60–9.

32. Dazzi F, Tarsitani L, Di Nunzio M, Trincia V, Scifoni G, Ducci G. Psychopathological assessment of risk of restraint in acute psychiatric patients. J Nerv Ment Dis. 2017;205:458–65.
33. Soyka M, Ufer S. [Aggressiveness in schizophrenia: prevalence, psychopathological and sociodemographic correlates]. Fortschr Neurol Psychiatr. 2002;70:171–7.
34. Swanson JW, Holzer CE, Ganju VK, Jono RT. Violence and psychiatric disorder in the community: evidence from the epidemiologic catchment area surveys. Hosp Community Psychiatry. 1990;41:761–70.
35. Dean K, Walsh E, Morgan C, Demjaha A, Dazzan P, Morgan K, et al. Aggressive behaviour at first contact with services: findings from the AESOP first episode psychosis study. Psychol Med. 2007;37:547–57.
36. Monahan J, Appelbaum P. Reducing violence risk: diagnostically based clues from the MacArthur violence risk assessment study. In: Hodgins S, editor. Violence among the mentally ill. Dordrecht: Springer International Publishing; 2000.
37. Voyer P, Verreault R, Azizah GM, Desrosiers J, Champoux N, Bédard A. Prevalence of physical and verbal aggressive behaviours and associated factors among older adults in long-term care facilities. BMC Geriatr. 2005;5:13.
38. Paveza GJ, Cohen D, Eisdorfer C, Freels S, Semla T, Ashford JW, et al. Severe family violence and Alzheimer's disease: prevalence and risk factors. Gerontologist. 1992;32:493–7.
39. Marshall WL, Christie MM. Pedophilia and aggression. Crim Justice Behav. 1981;8:145–58.
40. Glick AR. The role of serotonin in impulsive aggression, suicide, and homicide in adolescents and adults: a literature review. Int J Adolesc Med Health. 2015;27:143–50.
41. Dazzi F, Scicchitano C. Neurotrasmettitori: differenze di genere. Riv Psichiatr. 2014;49:227–34.
42. Çetin F, Torun Y, Guney E. The role of serotonin in aggression and impulsiveness, serotonin. In: Shad K, editor. A chemical. London: IntechOpen; 2017.
43. Sachdev P, Kruk J. Restlessness: the anatomy of a neuropsychiatric symptom. Aust N Z J Psychiatry. 1996;30:38–53.
44. Dazzi F, Orso L, Picardi A, Biondi M. Psychopathological dimensions in emergency psychiatry: determinants of admission, compulsory treatment, and therapeutic intervention. In: Dimensional psychopathology. Berlin: Springer International Publishing; 2018. p. 159–74.
45. Dazzi F, Picardi A, Orso L, Biondi M. Predictors of inpatient psychiatric admission in patients presenting to the emergency department: the role of dimensional assessment. Gen Hosp Psychiatry. 2015;37:587–94.
46. Picardi A, Viroli C, Tarsitani L, Miglio R, de Girolamo G, Dell'Acqua G, et al. Heterogeneity and symptom structure of schizophrenia. Psychiatry Res. 2012;198:386–94.

Neurobiology of Aggression and Violence

2

Francesco Saverio Bersani, Simone Mimun, and Roberto Delle Chiaie

2.1 Introduction

Aggression has been defined by Vitiello and Stoff as *"a behaviour deliberately aimed at inflicting physical damage to persons or property"* [1].

When approaching the issue of human aggression, it is important to consider that aggressive behaviours are also present in animals, and among animals they have a key role in social interaction and evolution of species [1, 2]. As reviewed by Vitiello and Stoff, seven subtypes of animal aggression with different phenomenology and underlying biology can be identified: predatory, intermale, territorial, maternal, irritable, fear-induced, and instrumental [1]. Such subtypes of animal aggression can be further grouped in the two constructs of affective aggression, involving a state of hyperarousal and aimed at reacting to a perceived threat, and predatory aggression, involving a state of hypoarousal and aimed at securing a positive reward [1].

Similarly, the research on human aggression has led to the conceptualization of two qualitatively different types often identified as impulsive/defensive/affective aggression and non-impulsive/premeditated/offensive/predatory aggression [1, 3–5]. According to Siever, impulsive aggression *"is characterized by high levels of autonomic arousal and precipitation by provocation associated with negative emotions such as anger or fear"*, and *"it usually represents a response to a perceived stress"*, while premeditated aggression is *"a planned behavior that is not typically associated with frustration or response to immediate threat [...] is not invariably accompanied by autonomic arousal and is planned with clear goals in mind"* [3]. The recently introduced Research Domain Criteria include aggression also in the domain of frustrative non-reward, as a consequence of studies suggesting that aggression occurs after repeated, failed attempts to obtain rewards [4]. Additional classifications of human aggression include the distinction between physical,

F. S. Bersani (✉) · S. Mimun · R. Delle Chiaie
Department of Human Neurosciences, Sapienza University of Rome, Rome, Italy
e-mail: francescosaverio.bersani@uniroma1.it; r.dellechiaie@centrokahlbaum.it

© Springer Nature Switzerland AG 2021
M. Biondi et al. (eds.), *Empathy, Normalization and De-escalation*,
https://doi.org/10.1007/978-3-030-65106-0_2

verbal, and indirect aggression (respectively implying physical, verbal, and psychological harm), and the dichotomy between normal and abnormal aggression [2]; according to Haller, *"human aggression is considered abnormal if it violates moral and legal rules or if is associated with psychopathologic conditions"* [2].

Meloy has provided for forensic purposes a summary of the core features of affective and predatory violence [5]. According to the author, affective violence is characterized, among the other things, by intense autonomic arousal, subjective experience of emotion, reactive and immediate violence, internal or external perceived threat, threat reduction as the main goal, possible displacement of target, time-limited behavioural sequences, precedent public posturing, primarily emotional/defensive nature, and diffuse heightened awareness [5]; on the other hand, predatory violence is characterized, among the other things, by minimal or absent autonomic arousal, lack of conscious emotion, planned or purposeful violence, no imminent perceived threat, no displacement of target, behavioural sequences not limited in time, precedent private rituals, primarily attack nature, and focused heightened awareness [5].

Of relevance for research and clinical practice, while aggressive behaviours can occur in patients with psychiatric disorders, (1) they do not occur exclusively among subjects with mental disorders, and (2) within individuals with a psychiatric diagnosis, they are not specific of a single disorder, but rather they represent a dimension which spans traditional diagnostic boundaries [6, 7]. It has been reported that antisocial personality disorders, borderline personality disorders, conduct disorders, delirium, dementia, dissociative disorders, intermittent explosive disorders, mental retardation, oppositional defiant disorders, post-traumatic stress disorders, schizophrenia, and substance use disorders are psychiatric conditions associated with violence [8]. Consistently, our research team has recently used the SVARAD (acronym for the Italian name "Scala per la VAlutazione Rapida Dimensionale", i.e. rapid dimensional assessment scale) to evaluate 846 inpatients consecutively recruited at the Psychiatry Unit of Policlinico Umberto I Hospital, finding that the level of anger/aggressiveness was not markedly different across patients with heterogeneous psychiatric diagnoses [6].

2.2   Genetic and Molecular Underpinnings of Human Aggression

As recently reviewed by Veroude et al., (1) twin studies suggest that around 50% of the variance in aggressiveness may be attributable to genetic effects, and (2) candidate-gene studies and genome-wide association studies have preliminarily identified potential susceptibility genes for aggressive behaviours mainly related to dopaminergic and serotonergic systems [4]. A renowned case related to the genetic of aggression has been described by Brunner et al.: the authors analysed a kindred in which several males were affected by a syndrome of borderline mental retardation and abnormal behaviour which included impulsive aggression, arson, attempted rape, and exhibitionism, finding that each of five affected males showed a point mutation in the eighth exon of the monoamine oxidase A (MAOA) structural gene

[9]. Gene-environment interactions are considered relevant in the aetiology of aggressive behaviours, with data suggesting that subjects with genetic risk may be vulnerable to the effect of environmental factors (e.g. traumatic, social, cultural, interpersonal factors) in leading to increased levels of aggression [3, 6].

At the molecular level, several mediators have been linked to aggression, including serotonin, dopamine, norepinephrine, acetylcholine, glutamate, gamma-aminobutyric acid (GABA), vasopressin, oxytocin, opiates, cytokines, testosterone, and cortisol [3, 10].

Among the neurotransmitters, attention has been paid to the dopamine/serotonin interaction in the prefrontal cortex, with reduced serotonergic function and increased dopaminergic function being associated with increases in aggressive behaviours [11], and to the balance between glutamate and GABA, with reduced GABAergic function and increased glutamatergic function being associated with increases in aggressive behaviours [3]. An involvement of such neurotransmitters in the pathophysiology of aggression is indirectly supported by the evidence that certain psychiatric medications acting on the modulation of their activity (e.g. benzodiazepines, antipsychotics, mood stabilizers, selective serotonin reuptake inhibitors) have shown some effectiveness in decreasing levels of aggressiveness [3, 6, 8].

Among the studies on molecular mediators of aggression different from neurotransmitters, the role of testosterone has been extensively investigated. The research on the relationship between testosterone and aggression in humans has mainly been stimulated by studies suggesting that (1) in several animal species, testosterone facilitates aggression; (2) testosterone is higher in men than in women, with men having higher levels of aggression than women; and (3) individuals with more aggressive behaviours have higher levels of testosterone [12–14]. However, a causal relationship between these two phenomena has not been established, with several contradictory findings emerging on the issue which have recently been summarized by Haller: *"(1): females readily show aggressiveness despite their low testosterone levels; (2) aggression is not increased at puberty when testosterone levels increase; (3) high- and low-aggression individuals do not consistently differ in serum testosterone; (4) aggression does not increase in hypogonadal males when exogenous testosterone is administered to support sexual activity; (5) castration or antiandrogen administration to males is not associated with a consistent decrease in aggression; and (6) the replication of positive findings is often difficult"* [14].

Interesting, although preliminary, data are emerging which suggest a relationship between inflammation and aggression. In relation to this, Coccaro et al. recently found that (1) among individuals with personality disorders, C-reactive protein (CRP) is associated with higher scores of trait aggression and hostility [15], (2) levels of CRP and interleukin 6 are significantly higher in individuals with intermittent explosive disorder than in non-aggressive individuals with a psychiatric disorders and in non-aggressive individuals without history of a psychiatric disorder [16], and (3) individuals with intermittent explosive disorder have differently methylated CpG sites involved in the inflammatory/immune system compared to controls [17]. While the study of the role of inflammation in aggressive behaviour is still in its infancy, such evidence adds to the accumulating data indicating a prominent role on inflammatory response for behaviour and psychiatric conditions [18].

2.3   Neurophysiological Underpinnings
of Human Aggression

At the brain circuitry level, aggressive behaviour is thought to result from impaired complex relationships between cortical and sub-cortical structures, and more specifically between frontal and limbic systems [3], although several models on neural circuits subserving aggression have been proposed and are currently under investigation [19, 20]. A renowned illustration of the role of frontal cortex in the pathophysiology of aggression is the case of Phineas Gage (1823–1860): after an iron bar incidentally passed through his head damaging prefrontal regions, he experienced a significant change in personality and behaviour which also included increased impulsivity and reduced respect for social conventions [21].

A neurobiological pathway linking an emotional trigger to an aggressive behaviour has recently been described by Siever, and it involves three steps [3]. The first step includes the sensory processing of the stimulus/i; this step is thus potentially affected by primary sensory distortions (e.g. disorders characterized by impaired auditory or visual processing) or by sensory distortions secondary to external circumstances (e.g. medications, drugs) [3]. Consistently, use of alcohol, cannabis, cocaine, methamphetamines, opiates, and certain novel psychoactive substances has been found associated with increased aggressive behaviours [22, 23]. The second step includes the appraisal and evaluation of the perceived stimulus/i; such evaluation can be influenced by a range of individual psychobiological characteristics, such as previous exposition to traumatic experiences, cultural and social factors, salience, as well as disturbances in thought (e.g. psychotic disorders) and in cognition (e.g. neurocognitive disorders) [3]. In relation to this, a relevant role is played by resilience, with studies suggesting that coping strategies influence individual responses to social stress, thus contributing to modulate aggressive behaviours [24]. The last step includes the activation of bottom-up limbic-frontal stimuli (emotional activation), which are usually counterbalanced by top-down fronto-limbic stimuli (executive functioning, planning, control of behaviours with potential negative consequences): an imbalance in such circuitry, with the bottom-up emotional response being stronger than the top-down control response, may result in aggressive behaviours [3]. This is consistent with evidence suggesting that lesions in frontal areas (e.g. related to neurodegenerative, traumatic, vascular or neoplastic mechanisms) are associated with increased violence [6, 8]. Of relevance, it has been pointed out that disturbances in executive functioning processes are more closely related to reactive aggression than to proactive aggression [10].

2.4   Conclusion

In conclusion, a growing amount of data is providing insight into the biological underpinnings of aggressiveness, at the ethological, genetic, molecular, and physiological level. Further studies are needed to better elucidate pathophysiological mechanisms and to transfer the findings to clinical practice.

References

1. Vitiello B, Stoff DM. Subtypes of aggression and their relevance to child psychiatry. J Am Acad Child Adolesc Psychiatry. 1997;36(3):307–15.
2. Haller J. Normal and abnormal aggressions: definitions and operational approaches. In: Neurobiological bases of abnormal aggression and violent behaviour. Wien: Springer; 2014. p. 1–31.
3. Siever LJ. Neurobiology of aggression and violence. Am J Psychiatry. 2008;165(4):429–42.
4. Veroude K, et al. Genetics of aggressive behavior: an overview. Am J Med Genet B Neuropsychiatr Genet. 2016;171B(1):3–43.
5. Meloy JR. Empirical basis and forensic application of affective and predatory violence. Aust N Z J Psychiatry. 2006;40(6–7):539–47.
6. Bersani FS, Pasquini M. The "outer dimensions": impulsivity, anger/aggressiveness, activation. In: Biondi M, Pasquini M, Picardi A, editors. Dimensional psychopathology. Cham: Springer International Publishing; 2018. p. 211–32.
7. Carpiniello B, Mencacci C, Vita A. Violence as a social, clinical, and forensic problem. In: Carpiniello B, Vita A, Mencacci C, editors. Violence and mental disorders. Cham: Springer Nature; 2020. p. 3–24.
8. Petit JR. Management of the acutely violent patient. Psychiatr Clin North Am. 2005;28(3):701–11, 710.
9. Brunner HG, et al. Abnormal behavior associated with a point mutation in the structural gene for monoamine oxidase A. Science. 1993;262(5133):578–80.
10. Manchia M, et al. Neurobiology of violence. In: Carpiniello B, Vita A, Mencacci C, editors. Violence and mental disorders. Cham: Springer Nature; 2020. p. 25–47.
11. Seo D, Patrick CJ, Kennealy PJ. Role of serotonin and dopamine system interactions in the neurobiology of impulsive aggression and its comorbidity with other clinical disorders. Aggress Violent Behav. 2008;13(5):383–95.
12. Wong JS, Gravel J. Do sex offenders have higher levels of testosterone? Results from a meta-analysis. Sex Abuse. 2018;30(2):147–68.
13. Archer J. The influence of testosterone on human aggression. Br J Psychol. 1991;82(Pt 1):1–28.
14. Haller J. Hormonal determinants. In: Neurobiological bases of abnormal aggression and violent behaviour. Wien: Springer; 2014. p. 33–68.
15. Coccaro EF. Association of C-reactive protein elevation with trait aggression and hostility in personality disordered subjects: a pilot study. J Psychiatr Res. 2006;40(5):460–5.
16. Coccaro EF, Lee R, Coussons-Read M. Elevated plasma inflammatory markers in individuals with intermittent explosive disorder and correlation with aggression in humans. JAMA Psychiat. 2014;71(2):158–65.
17. Montalvo-Ortiz JL, et al. Genome-wide DNA methylation changes associated with intermittent explosive disorder: a gene-based functional enrichment analysis. Int J Neuropsychopharmacol. 2018;21(1):12–20.
18. Halaris A, Leonard BE. Inflammation in psychiatry. Basel: Karger International; 2013.
19. Haller J. Neural circuits subserving aggression: general models. In: Neurobiological bases of abnormal aggression and violent behaviour. Wien: Springer; 2014. p. 69–78.
20. Haller J. Focal points of aggression control. In: Neurobiological bases of abnormal aggression and violent behaviour. Wien: Springer; 2014. p. 79–144.
21. Damasio H, et al. The return of Phineas Gage: clues about the brain from the skull of a famous patient. Science. 1994;264(5162):1102–5.
22. Tomlinson MF, Brown M, Hoaken PNS. Recreational drug use and human aggressive behavior: a comprehensive review since 2003. Aggress Violent Behav. 2016;27:9–29.
23. Schifano F, et al. Substance-use disorders and violence. In: Carpiniello B, Vita A, Mencacci C, editors. Violence and mental disorders. Cham: Springer Nature; 2020. p. 95–114.
24. Veenema AH, Neumann ID. Neurobiological mechanisms of aggression and stress coping: a comparative study in mouse and rat selection lines. Brain Behav Evol. 2007;70:274–85.

Empathy Regulation in Crisis Scenario

3

Martina Valentini, Irene Pinucci, and Massimo Pasquini

3.1 Introduction

The ability to know how to speak to a person who is afraid, angry, depressed, aggressive and delusional or who has received bad news about their physical health is not an innate skill but should be learned and integrate as a professional skill. In difficult or emergency situations, knowing how to communicate empathically with a person can in many cases resolve the situation or improve it greatly, increasing patient compliance and collaboration and avoiding the act of aggressive actions towards the healthcare professional as much as possible. But the empathic communication is not an innate skill and requires to act not symmetrically to the patient's emotional state; this is a skill that can be learned and perfected with practice. In particular, it's crucial to know *what* (verbal aspects of communication) to say and *how* (non-verbal aspects of communication) to say it.

Before starting and engaging in a communication in emergency situation, the healthcare professional needs to have a "map" to orientate in the communication and keep control of the situation (Table 3.1).

According to our communication model, empathic communication is the first step to actualize, followed by normalization and de-escalation. Based on the situation that has to be faced, sometimes the clinician practices more a technique than another (e.g. when the patient is angry and possibly aggressive, there's more need do communicate in an empathic way and use more de-escalation rather than normalization), but in general, all the three types of communication are used during a communication in difficult or emergency situations.

In this chapter, we present the fundamentals of empathy, its biological roots, the way to actualize empathic communication followed by case vignettes to better

M. Valentini (✉) · I. Pinucci · M. Pasquini
Department of Human Neurosciences, Faculty of Medicine and Dentistry,
SAPIENZA University of Rome, Rome, Italy
e-mail: martina.valentini@uniroma1.it

© Springer Nature Switzerland AG 2021
M. Biondi et al. (eds.), *Empathy, Normalization and De-escalation*,
https://doi.org/10.1007/978-3-030-65106-0_3

Table 3.1 Conceptual map of the elements to keep in mind before starting the empathic communication

What?	Before engaging in a communication with a patient/person, think of what to say, that is, the precise content you want to communicate, e.g. that you recognize and understand the underlying emotional state of the other one or that you recognize that for the other one it's a very difficult situation. In empathic communication, it's crucial to communicate the other one that his emotional state is well recognized
To who?	Who is the person we are going to talk to? Is it an angry, aggressive, scared or depressed patient or a family member or a significant other? The empathic communication must be modulated according to who we are facing
When?	At what moment? Is it better to wait for a while or begin immediately the empathic communication?
How?	Choose the exact words to use in that situation according to the emotional, mental and physical state of the person you are facing. This is one of the most important points in empathic communication (and in general in END communication), and as we will further see, there are sentences that can be learned and trained that communicate that you have recognized and understood the emotional/mental state of the other one
Where?	Where is the communication happening (or will happen)? The patient is lying in bed in a hospital ward, or in a room with other persons, waiting room, emergency department, etc. Where possible, try to choose a quiet place in which empathic communication can be done at best
To which people?	Are there other people the patient wants to be? For example, family members, partner, friend, etc. Probably, in cases where anger and aggressiveness are present, the more persons are around, the more the sanitary will feel under attack; this is important to figure out, because this will probably make the empathic communication more difficult to be implemented
How to talk	Based on the situation to addressed, choose the tone of the voice, the facial expressions, the body movements, the distance and all the non-verbal aspects of communication. This is another crucial point for empathic communication, because non-verbal aspects can be captured on a very deep level by the patient
Verify	At the end of the empathic communication, verify what effect that type of communication had on the patient. In particular, check if the other one has understood that we have recognized his emotional state in that moment

explain the difference between empathic communication and good/bad communication (i.e. all that communications that are not specific to gain the relationship with the other person). We even describe the importance of non-verbal communication as a part of empathic communication, another skill to learn and improve in clinical/professional settings.

3.2 Definition

Empathy has had a lot of definitions in philosophy, human sciences, psychology and psychiatry as well as in general medicine.

The etymological route of empathy is the German term "Einfühlung", literally "sich ausweisen", that is "identify themselves" [1]. It was originally introduced in the aesthetic theory of Vischer [2] and Lipps [3], explaining the experience of beauty and art as a profound consonance between object and subject. Empathy was then introduced in psychology, psychiatry and psychotherapy, as well as in medicine, and is a component of the therapeutic relationship and care, with a careful distinction from sympathy (i.e. syn "together" and pathos "suffering"). Empathy was a basic notion in the field of psychoanalysis and humanistic psychotherapy, with a contribution of several other authors. The conception of "Einfühlung" of Freud was traced in the paper "Der Witz und seine Beziehung zum Umbewussten" [4], and he considered "Einfühlung" (which was not exactly translated as "empathy" in English) pivotal for the relationship between the analysts and the patients [1]. A seminal work was done by Norma Feshbach with her studies on the development of empathy and empathic behaviour in children [5]. Contemporary position suggests multiple forms of empathy, such as the cognitive empathy (Theory of Mind), the motor empathy and the emotional empathy. They are not rigidly separated but do share areas of anatomical and functional overlap [6].

Several psychometric scales for the measurement of empathy are available in literature, such as Jefferson Scale of Empathy. The JSE is probably the most widely used instrument, which has translation in 55 different countries, and is mainly used in healthcare settings. In a study in which a factor analysis was conducted, the author found four main factors with the following labels: (1) "Physicians view from the patients perspective"; (2) "Understanding patients experiences, feelings and clues"; (3) "Ignoring emotions in patients"; and (4) "Thinking like the patient" [7].

After being at the centre of human psychology and ethology studies, conceived as one of the prosocial behaviours [8], in recent years empathy has become an interesting issue for the neurosciences, with several studies of brain imaging correlates of empathy processes [9].

As fully emphasized by Heyes from the Department of Experimental Psychology, University of Oxford, "Empathy is [...] a psychological phenomenon, rooted in biology, with profound effects in law, policy, and international relations. But the roots of empathy are not as firm as we like to think [...]. Research with animals, infants, adults and robots suggests that the mechanism of Empathy, emotional contagion, is constructed in the course of development through social interaction. Learned Matching implies that empathy is both agile and fragile. It can be enhanced and redirected by novel experience, and broken by social change" [10].

So, this means that empathic thinking and communication are not innate but can be learned and developed with specific techniques and that empathic communication is a skill. In common diplomacy, common interpersonal relationships, work relation and medical settings, empathic communication is not an automatic skill, but it requests a specific "attitude" to begin with. To put oneself in attitude means in our model and point of view to make the effort to act in a non-conflictual way, empty the mind and be goal centred; focus on the main points and techniques prior a difficult communication with a patient; to have a communicate "respect for the patient", let them feel considerate; don't feign: the ability to communicate is a professional tool that can be learned. Furthermore, the empathic communication skills implicate the rapid ability to represent the other one's mental state and to wait some seconds prior to answer, producing a firmly answer that searches for a meeting point using expressions like "we" and not "you and I"; while we use the END communication procedure, we have to pay attention to our tone of voice. Since empathic communication is a learned skill, making part of the professional skills, it means that if someone is verbally offended and mistreated, then it is not recommended to answer at the same "emotional level" (escalation), as it would naturally happen. In a healthcare setting (like many other settings), one should have a professional role, defending oneself from verbal offenses and mistreating without counterattacking, except of a physical aggression. If possible, take some time to think and to answer using END communication.

In this chapter, we will define "empathy" as an operationalized concept based on recognition of other one's feelings, emotions and sensations and verbal restitution in a comprehensive and interacting way.

According to the Theory of Mind (ToM) [11], a person can recognize a mental state of another one, attributing him beliefs, feelings and intentions, with a set of specific brain network dedicated to the task. Empathy can be also considered a type of social cognition, where the recognition of emotions is centred. In our view, empathy is conceived not only as an ability of inferring and representing the other one's mental state but also all the interpersonal procedures and expressions given in a reciprocal and mutual communication. In this way, our use of the term empathy is more operational than theoretical. It can be translated, as we will further explain, in two subsequent steps: (1) the ability of recognizing, of intuition, and of hypothesizing the mental state and the predominant feelings, given a specific situation and circumstances (i.e. of a patient at the moment of a hospital admission or emergency situations), and (2) the act of communicating to the person in a formal way the hypothesized state of mind, suggesting that the speaker has recognized and understood the other one's feelings and state of mind.

The further exploration of other's feelings leads to the process of empathic communication.

The empathic communication establishes a "bridge" with the other person, and it opens the way to the second step, the normalization process, and to the third step, the de-escalation and negotiation communication.

3.3 Neural Bases of Empathy

The nature of emphatic sharing is complex, and several factors determined its process such as the sense of belonging to the proper family, the sense of place and also the sense of ethnical, political or professional identity. Human survival was due to the ability of emphatic sharing. In this sense, what happens to our brain when we put ourselves in the shoes of the person who is talking to us? Which parts of our grey matters are activated when we comprehend, share and feel what we are hearing and seeing? To which neuronal pathways should we address when we are trying to reach an empathic communication? Starting from the end of the 1980s, research has focused on neuronal basis of empathy, suggesting a neuronal firing in temporal lobe in response to somatic mimicry of other primates at the basis of empathy functions and conferring an evolutionary role to the ability to understand and empathize with our communicators [12].

The *social brain hypothesis* is the result of an anthropological research around the dimensions reached by brains in primates compared to other vertebrates, with a particular role of the neocortex. This last one would indeed be the main responsible for the expansion of the primate brain due to the "ability to manipulate information about social relationships" [13]. Coping with complex social lives and cognitive demands of bonds (which for primates are extended to friends, a new kind of relationship that goes beyond the procreational role) would explain such dimensions [14], together with the ability to make predictions about actions accomplished by others [15] and to cooperate to obtain food and ensuring offspring [16]. Different cerebral regions were described as involved in specific roles: while the amygdala would underpin associations of values to people and objects, regulating social behaviour and recognizing emotional facial expression, the temporal pole (TP) would be able to discern knowledge about a specific social situation from a general acquaintance, the posterior superior temporal sulcus (pSTS) would predict movement trajectories, the temporoparietal junction (TPJ) would let us understand that a person has a false belief (as in the Sally-Anne task described later), the medial prefrontal cortex (MPFC) would make us understand what is our communicator's perception of our own mental state and predict the value of our actions towards other people, and finally the orbitofrontal cortex would be involved in reward processing while the insula in representing states such as pain proved by our body or by someone else [13, 14].

The fundamental evolutionary role attributed to social brain leads us to wonder how we can read others' emotion and thoughts. In order to answer to this question, numerous researches focused their attention on those conditions causing an empathic dysfunction including mental diseases, personality disorders, autism and morphological alterations.

Psychopathic individuals, as a paradigmatic example of a lack of empathy, were largely studied. Having a conversation with a psychopathic individual can represent a tricky challenge due to the pervasive feeling of communicating with somebody whose feelings fly far beyond our preoccupations. Dysfunctions in the amygdala and ventromedial prefrontal cortex were described as a cause of their reactive and instrumental aggression caused by an emotion dysfunction [17–20]. Empathy dysfunctions were also studied in *schizophrenic patients*, still proposing a fundamental role of amygdala together with temporal and orbitofrontal cortex and suggesting a dysfunction of the interaction between social cognition (frontal lobes) and their functionally connected cortical and subcortical areas [21]. Concerning *autism*, an empathy dysfunction, would affect many domains, and it was proposed that it could even represent the principal cause of every different clinical autistic feature [22, 23]. Finally, it was observed that *morphological alterations* of brain structure can represent a cause of a modification of empathic functions. The famous clinical case of Phineas Gage described by Harlow [24], the railroad employee whose frontal lobes was penetrated by an iron bar provoking marked modifications in social behaviour, can be considered one of the first described examples of an altered empathic response caused by a cerebral lesion. The role of PFC was confirmed by more recent studies describing empathy deficits as a consequence of a brain damage [25].

But what kind of empathy are we considering when we talk about neuronal basis of empathic functions? Many different definitions were given to this multifaceted concept [26], but two of them mostly took into consideration when focusing on neurobiological bases of emphatic functions: cognitive empathy and emotional empathy [27, 28].

Cognitive empathy would be involved in reflective processes producing a representation of the mental states of other people referable to the Theory of Mind (ToM) [29, 30], well explained by the Sally-Anne task, where the participant is asked to represent a doll's mental state about where a marble is after showing him that it was moved from its original position during doll's absence [31, 32]. ToM's function can be investigated by the "Advanced Theory of Mind test" [33] and the "Reading the Mind in the Eyes" task [34], originally developed to study adults with autism and Asperger syndrome. We have already mentioned the critical role of an empathic dysfunction within the autism spectrum, and both of these tests show an impaired function for individuals with autism.

Emotional empathy represents the act of sharing feelings and affective states showed by another person, and it was recently described as composed by two main different psychological processes: emotional empathy (which would involve the amygdala, insula, somatosensory cortex) and empathic concern, also called compassion (which would involve the periaqueductal grey, hypothalamus, striatum and ventromedial prefrontal cortex) [35].

Interestingly, psychopathic individuals seem to present a normal ToM's function [36–38], while an impaired cognitive empathy accompanied by preserved functions of emotional empathy seems to be presented by patients with schizophrenia [39, 40].

Two different neural routes, highlighted using functional magnetic resonance imaging (fMRI), would underpin them: the anterior insula (AI), anterior cingulate/ dorsomedial prefrontal cortex (ACC/dmPFC), posterior cingulate cortex (PCC), rostral anterior cingulate cortex (rACC), anterior midcingulate cortex (aMCC), inferior frontal gyrus (IFG), dorsal portions of the temporoparietal junction/supramarginal gyrus (TPJ/SMG), supplementary motor area (SMA), midbrain, left anterior thalamus, amygdala (AM), middle temporal gyrus (MTG), posterior superior temporal sulcus (pSTS), posterior thalamus, hippocampus and right pallidum were described as involved in processes underpinning *emotional empathy*, while *ToM-related networks* would involve the TPJ (considered the core network of ToM), medial prefrontal cortex (mPFC), superior temporal gyrus/sulcus (STG/STS), precuneus (Prec), temporal poles (TP), pSTS, middle temporal gyrus (MTG), IFG and right middle temporal visual area (MT) [41–43].

Volumetric differences of cerebral regions would be involved in the effectiveness of both empathic functions, as they were proposed by studies that focused on individual differences in grey matters density measured through a voxel-based morphometry (VBM). It was demonstrated that a larger bilateral grey density in the insula and in midcingulate cortex (MCC) and adjacent dorsomedial prefrontal cortex (dmPFC) would be associated with higher scores on the affective empathy scale and the cognitive empathy scale, respectively [44].

Recently, a new behavioural and fMRI paradigm was developed called *EmpaToM*. Its function is to study cerebral and behavioural markers related to empathy and compassion, focusing on whether the neuronal activity observed during empathic functions could be related to empathy ratings but not to Tom's ones and vice versa. Different neural networks were demonstrated respectively for empathy and ToM, together with an increased activation of neural networks in response to an enhanced performance for each of the two domains. Moreover, specific peaks were identified in overlapping regions (involving TPJ and precuneus/posterior cingulate mPFC which would present a more ventral peak for ToM and a dorsal one for empathic functions) [45]. The generalizability of empathy and ToM-related neural activity and the reproducibility of EmpaToM were recently confirmed across subject- and item-wise analyses [41].

This clear separation between emotional and cognitive empathy is still a topic of discussion; indeed some authors highlight the overestimation of their distinction and the risk to repeat a dichotomization between science and philosophy [46, 47]. Although extremely interesting, such epistemological controversy goes beyond the scopes of these pages.

Moreover, a third empathic response called *motor empathy* was proposed, based upon the *mirror function* described for some neurons capable of creating a communication between perception and movement. When observing a goal-directed action, mirror neurons respond as if the subject was acting himself, suggesting a role in mediating understanding of actions done by others [48–52]. Empathizing with others' emotions, or mirror-matching them, would represent the instrument to understand them [53]. It was proposed that this mechanism could be involved in the empathic comprehension of an emotional state, which would determine a corresponding representation in the observer through a neuronal automatic activation that establishes a perception-action model (PAM) [54]. Differences between the mirror neuron system and PAM however were described by the same authors of PAM theory, illustrating this last one as focusing more on "distributed representations that include relevant feelings, memories and associations that are related to the target, and to the target's state and situation" [46].

Besides neuronal firing, also neurochemical differences underpinning these two different empathic domains were detected: *oxytocin*, the most abundant neuropeptide of the hypothalamus, would be more involved in emotional empathy enhancing the detection of positive facial expressions [55] and socially reinforced learning [56]. In the light of these findings, intranasal oxytocin administration was tested as a mean to increase empathic functions with success in specific populations [57–59], albeit not all studied populations confirmed these results [60]. Modulatory effects of this neuropeptide on the amygdala were suggested [61].

Another pivotal issue is if and how empathic response could be modulated? The affective link between two people, gender, personality and age seems to have a role in this modulation, and regulation mechanisms related to appraisal processes, also at a subpersonal level, were proposed [62]. Moreover, empathic brain responses would be modulated by empathy traits evaluated through self-report questionnaires or by state measures of felt empathic concern, and an antagonistic motivation to empathy would be related to feelings of revenge [63]. Besides the activation of areas involved in cognitive, emotional or motor empathy through a bottom-up process, top-down mechanisms of control of human empathy were described, determining a flexibility of the empathic reaction based on the ability of attention, context appraisal and perspective-taking [64]. A voluntary control over the mechanisms involved in empathizing was recently described, involving a modulated activation of limbic and somatomotor regions, the same involved in mirror neuron functions [65]. The same study showed that modulating empathy has an impact on how we report the perception of other's people feelings.

When we are trying to reach an empathic communication, we use the described empathic functions to imagine and depict the internal status of out communicator. Such functions represent an indispensable tool to communicate with a psychiatric patient. Moreover, modulating them has a crucial role for multiple reasons: first, dampening emotional empathic functions could represent an instrument to safeguard health workers from an excessive emotional involvement. Mental health workers showed enhanced empathy skills compared to general physicians and non-medical workers associated with more frequent experiences of preoccupations and uneasiness related to empathizing. Years of experience in mental health works showed to modulate scores in empathic domain, and a progressive desensitization to mental suffering was proposed as an explanation for this phenomenon. Besides, empathic skills seem to be modifiable by external factors such as workplace type and moral judgement in mental health workers [66].

Second, modulation of patient's empathic functions could have consequences for different fundamental abilities. It was indeed recently proposed that empathy could be involved in the *insight* abilities in psychiatric disorders. The same authors described a subjective (embodiment through the mirror neuron system and emotional processes) and an objective (ToM and self-regulatory processes of visuospatial perspective-taking) dimension of empathy, positing that the process of objectification (cognitive recognition the presented disease) is an indispensable condition for the correct evolution of the process subjectification (the incorporation of the other's point of view in the representation of the self) and so therefore for the insight functions [66]. Such theory would confirm what is frequently experienced when trying to reach an empathic communication with patients: altered empathic functions would determine a hard communication due to the impaired ability to tune with the communicator toughened by the weak insight functions.

3.4 Empathic Communication and Its Mechanism of Action

In our model, empathy is defined as "empathic communication" with some specific aims: the first aim is to let the other one feel that "I understand" and "I recognize pain, suffering, preoccupation, feelings of fear and helplessness/hopelessness"; the second aim is to communicate or better "transmit" that I understand that the other one is probably perceiving the present situation and that "you can see from his/her point of view"; the third aim is that you can represent his/her mental state and without judgement the emotions that are running on and that I am in tune with these experiencing.

One of the points for the intervention in the psychiatric field is to move towards a diagnostic framework according to a profile of predominant psychopathological dimensions and by area rather than by research of an exact diagnostic category, in other words, if a person is overwhelmed by fear, or delusions, or shows aggressive behaviour, we will try to communicate with them by treating these aspects first, making it possible to implement subsequent therapeutic actions (e.g. voluntary admission, pharmacological therapy, etc.). Our method therefore identifies the most critical condition at which to focus attention and intervention: using the dimensional approach, by creating dimensional profiles of suffering, helps even to identify the brain areas and circuits involved in a critical situation and which are the target of the communication. In particular, empathic communication "talks" to the limbic system of the other person, in order to "calm it down" and prepare the field for the frontal cortex (using normalization and de-escalation).

The final aim of empathic communication is to build a bridge between "you" and the other person, which represents the first step for the further subsequent phases of normalization and de-escalation.

In our procedure, empathic communication is *not* intended to give someone reason, give a comment and not take side but only to communicate that we understand how the other one is feeling and that we are by his/her side, letting them know that we are there for them and deeply understanding what is humanly going on. Empathic communication is not reassuring; reassurance is possible only after you have explored, listened and assessed, that is, at the end of the communication process.

Some good but not empathic phrases or expressions are not empathic (see Table 3.2).

Table 3.2 Examples of "good" but *not* empathic phrases

"Be calm"	Examples of good, but not empathic phrases. These are examples of phrases that everyone, who is not trained in emphatic communication, could say (e.g. a friend, a parent)
"We will help you"	
"Don't worry"	
"Everything is under control"	
"Keep calm"	
"There is no reason to worry"	
"I'm here for you"	
"It happened to me too"	
"Don't think about it, it's nothing"	
"Everything will be alright"	

Case Vignette 1

M. is 60 years old, married and has two children who still depend on him. Recently he has had problems at work, feels stressed and knows he has altered blood chemistry parameters. He takes antihypertensive drugs and is worried about a slight pain he sometimes experiences at night in the chest area. So, he schedules an appointment with his cardiologist. The doctor welcomes him and listens to his anamnesis: he prepares to do some instrumental tests and approaches him saying: "Don't worry, it's nothing special. You only have to calm down".

Since the doctor knows they are fans of the same football team, he begins to talk to him about the team's latest games.

The patient actually remains worried and talks about football with discomfort because he thinks about his heart and thinks he has a heart attack. He feels that his feelings, fears and worries are ignored by the doctor. The reassurance of the cardiologist is not effective because it happens before the physical assessment and diagnostic procedures and is therefore not competent to exclude the diagnosis of disease. The cardiologist's intent to calm the patient is good-natured but not effective.

Case Vignette 2

A is 20 years old with a diagnosis of borderline personality disorder and enters the outpatient room for his visit with the young psychotherapist. He is openly tensed, restless and somewhat angry. His first words are: "It's your fault, I don't improve and things are getting worser. You're not able to do your job. You promised me I would get better, but you're a liar. I'm so angry with you, I would like to break something!"

The psychotherapist answers: "Oh come on, calm down! There is no reason to be angry … relax yourself, you have everything a person of your age could deserve. There is really no reason to react like this".

These words increase the patient's irritation, and he leaves and prematurely interrupts the session saying: "You don't understand me!"

The next day, during a session with his supervisor, the psychotherapist tells the difficulties encountered with this patient and attributes the interruption of the session to the patient's impulsiveness and to the ego's defensive ability to withstand a tension. His work plan was to focus on this while sitting with the patient. The supervisor explains that the patient is certainly impulsive, unstable and unable to self-regulate emotions but that the psychotherapist did not recognize the patient's emotion (who felt rejected) and probably felt the therapist's words as a judgement. This further increased the patient's anger.

While there are many treatises, articles and papers on the importance of empathy in medicine and psychotherapy, few provide specific and concrete procedures on how to implement empathic communication.

Empathic communication needs to face up other difficulties: scared, depressed and angry persons and patients, sometimes with reality distortion and other psychopathological symptoms that could represent an obstacle to communication, understanding and subsequent compliance for treatment. The main reason is that the active emotional state compromises the reception and elaboration of the messages in the usual way.

The first requirement is to recognize that the communication between health professionals and patients and the use of empathic communication is not a spontaneous way of communication but is a "professional tool" that needs to be learned, improved and perfected.

Therefore, the second requirement is that the person who is entering in a relationship with a patient in a difficult or emergency situation disposes himself in an attitude of empathic communication. This means to leave your own "emotional troubles", preoccupations and thoughts, like a surgeon does when he is about to operate, in empathic communication you have to concentrate on what to communicate, what to say and how to say it, balancing the tone of the voice, the mimic and the non-verbal communication and verifying the effects of the communication on the other person. Furthermore, as concerns aspects of non-verbal communication, we suggest do not stare directly, nor look elsewhere; do not touch the patient; keep the body in a natural and relaxed attitude; check the tone of voice (not too loud) and avoid that the tone of voice increases during a sentence; do not keep your arms tight; speak slowly and in short sentences; use one or two same words that the patient used to tune in; and leave spaces and silences (if necessary) without pressing. We also suggest training with your own recordings and listening to them several times to perfect the unsatisfactory points. When possible, it is useful to organize in the team, led by an expert conductor, simulations with the adult learning and practice-based learning techniques.

Before starting the empathic communication and enter in relation with the patient, there are some key points to remember: first of all, the health professional needs to prepare himself to assume an open and non-conflictual attitude towards the patient; to plan what to say and how to say it; and to clear the mind and point to the target, concentrating on the task; all these steps need to be figured out and prepared before engaging in an empathic communication with a patient in a difficult situation and where the emotional level is very high.

If possible, it should be important to collect information about the patient and medical/psychiatric history in order to better connect with the patient's issue.

A good attitude to communicate requires an unconditioned respect for the other person, and this should be an essential property of a healthcare professional.

Empathic communication is synthetic, uses few words and is, as we will see, developed in a maximum of two sentences. To use a metaphor, empathic communication photographs, does not dilute the narrative and does not add comments or personal considerations but is only focused on the patient's mood and emotional activation and tries to reflect and give this feedback to the other person.

Finally, communication skills require the ability to communicate in an authentic way without pretending. The professional communication wants the healthcare professional to be genuine and not forced in the communication.

Prefer when you are exploring what and how questions rather than why questions, because the term "why" commonly leads to intellectualization, rationalization, automatic and justification answers. *What* and *how* questions, instead, are "open questions" and let the patients have the opportunity to report their feeling and thoughts. A key of the empathic communication is to talk "with the patient" and not "talk to the patient". In the commonest clinical situations with medical patients, there is no need of going to deep nor of giving explanations or interpretations, which can add unnecessary or difficult material. They can be explored and discussed in other specific settings. There is a difference between "reflecting" communications and furtherly adding communications. In the empathic communication, we should not suggest feelings, especially our own feelings in that given situation (this is a common error), but rely on your own clinical experience about what the feelings of *those* patients *in that specific* situation—you have observed—might be. The feelings and reactions could be different on the basis of age, gender, clinical history, etc.

As Walter Baile [67] suggested, it is necessary for the healthcare provider to have a map in his mind before having a contact with the patient: having a map means knowing where you want to go, what to ask for, what are the objectives and what could be in general the possible difficulties to be faced. To do this, the healthcare provider can concentrate, before coming into contact with the patient, on some crucial aspects of the subjective experience of the patient.

Crucial questions are: How can the patient feel right now? What do you know about his situation? What can most probably worry him most? Another question is: What answer has he found so far to his questions and issues? Finally, explore who he can count on next to him or as a support and reference?

As part of effective empathic communication, the healthcare professional can speak for just 1 min and ask him directly for the first point; for the second point, he can ask the patient "what idea he has of his ailment/problem"; as regards the third point, the best is to ask directly who are the significant one's next to him who can support the patient. Again, the fourth question to ask is what has been communicated to him by the other health professionals he has met; in reference to the fifth point, it's important to observe who is around the patient and who accompanies him and ask if there is someone he wants the physician or healthcare professional to talk to.

The third requirement is to use operationally specific sentences that actualize empathy. In this sense, according to our point of view, good but generic phrases like "Don't worry", "It's all right", "It's nothing serious" and "Don't worry" (Table 3.2) are not empathetic.

The procedures for empathic communication do not entail giving the patient reason, judging, commenting or reassuring in a generic way. Reassuring is not an empathic communication, although it can be useful, especially when it is done as an opening of the interview. The reassurance communication is valid only after it has been investigated and understood how the other person feels, for example, after completing a physical visit, after taking an anamnesis and after getting the results of laboratory data. With this knowledge in hand, reassurance will be felt as effective communication.

A central requirement of empathic communication is to try to identify the main emotion that the person can feel at that specific moment (phase 1) and to only communicate him to understand the way he feels.

The empathic communication requires to develop and train at best in a "surgical" precision of the words, as if they were a scalpel. The aim is that only precise words spoken in a reasoned way allow you to reach the established goal; you need to train a lot to get to a good degree of mastery that is learned over time after many attempts that are natural and simple.

Case Vignette 3

S. is hospitalized in a surgical clinic and will be operated tomorrow. The patient is in his bed and is very worried because they have told him that surgery is difficult for his case but must still be done to remove a tumour. During the informed consent procedure, they told him that there is risk of severe complications, they'll do everything to avoid them, but there's still some percentage of risk of death. A young surgeon enters the room and asks how he is while visiting him quickly. The patient says he is very worried, and his face shows marked anguish. The doctor says to him in a ringing voice: "No no, don't worry, everything will be fine. Come on, tomorrow night there is the final game and we will win the championship". And goes away smiling.

In this example, the clinician probably tried to protect himself (unconsciously?) from the patient's strong and sad emotions, avoiding his own distress of an open communication about the issue; so the doctor gives a quick and superficial answer. The last comments of the doctor are an attempt to play down the difficult situation and divert attention, trying in his own way to give the charge. In reality, communication is a failure from the point of view of managing emotions. The patient does not feel understood; he remains worried and even humiliated by an answer that ignores his need.

This doesn't mean that the clinicians can't joke or be nice to the patients, but only after an actual empathic communication.

Based on what has been defined, therefore, the structure of an empathic sentence is articulated and fixed: the structure of the sentence includes recognizing the other person's main emotion and talking to him about it. As a rule, it is preferable to use

Table 3.3 Examples of empathic phrases that can be used in empathic communication

From what I understand, the last few days have been really difficult	These phrases tune in the emotional state of the other one and communicate that we understand the underlying emotion of the patient
This moment must be really hard for you	
I think you don't really want to talk to us right now	
It must be a bad experience for you to be here right now	
You might be worried about what is happening to you now	
I guess you're worried about what's happening to your wife	
With everything that happened, I think you are really angry	
Maybe you're a little scared now, can I help you?	
Maybe you are worried or scared about being observed here at the emergency room	

a doubtful or hypothetical form in the description of the prevailing emotional state. Useful terms are "perhaps" or "maybe" and below example phrases (Table 3.3):

- "Maybe you are scared now, can I help you?"
- "You will be worried about staying and being observed here in the hospital …"
- "Maybe you are very tired, you have been unable to sleep well for many days".

In other cases, explorative expressions can be used, like "It happened all so quickly; can you tell me how you feel?"

Case Vignette 4

C. is taken by ambulance and with the police to the emergency room. The patient is very agitated and aggressive, so much so that he has to be hospitalized in compulsory mode. When the psychiatrist consultant arrives at the emergency room, the patient is verbally violent, refuses all treatment and even to speak. The psychiatrist introduces himself in a calm voice and says: "It seems you are very, very angry. Maybe you feel like they forced you to come here … do you want to tell me what happened and why you are so angry?"; the patient looks at him a moment and after a few seconds starts speaking: "I was at home, I felt nervous because it's some nights that I can't sleep. My neighbours are angry with me, for days I have the voices that tell me and I shouted at them. They persecute me … in fact they called the police. At that point I was too angry".

The psychiatrist, after a moment, says, "I understand, it must be a really bad experience. You felt that the others spoke badly about you and everything fell so quickly".

The patient replies: "They took me by force and forced me to come here with an ambulance".

The psychiatrist says, "Being forced … makes you feel like you're losing your freedom. I'm sorry this happened to you".

The patient looks at the psychiatrist, is visibly calmer and is surprised to find someone who seems to understand him, and at that point, the psychiatrist says: "Let's talk about it. For many days you haven't slept, you're tired and nervous, let's see what we can do". In order to get some sleep and talk about what's going on with the neighbours, the patient will accept hospitalization. He even agrees that his psychiatrist who has been following him for months will also be called.

In many other cases, the healthcare professionals may encounter different difficult and emergency situations that the patient is living, like situations in which there's excessive physical pain, a patient receiving a breaking bad new and many other emotionally difficult situations that can be found in the clinical routine.

In all this cases, it is useful to start the communication whit a very simple sentence that expresses contact and recognition of the other one but that seems often so difficult to say for healthcare professionals and physicians; the simple phrase so difficult to enounce is "I feel sorry". For example, one could say: "I feel sorry that you are suffering from these pains, I feel sorry that the tests we are evaluating suggest problems to be addressed. I feel sorry for how you feel".

Communicating the phrase "I feel sorry" is difficult to say, and generally it is not done spontaneously because it communicates one's own personal mood and often the training of physicians and healthcare professionals teaches to be detached and impersonal. On the contrary, the phrase "I feel sorry" communicates a personal human openness towards the patient. Moreover, it is difficult to say because if the healthcare professional is witnessing something negative or painful that depends on medical/psychiatric/psychological situations, he/she can feel responsible and, at first, we tend to defend our self or to keep silent. The ability to say "sorry", which adds to empathic communication, is fundamental, if not decisive, when it comes to communicating medical errors. It involves a high emotional cost for the doctor who must recognize his mistake, face frustration and a sense of guilt, and that he has caused harm, even if not intentional, to the other person. Another example of the meaning of communicating to another person in an emphatic way is the communication of having done a mistake or a harm. The silence about professional mistakes and the avoidance of talking about it with the patient, explaining and communicating "I'm sorry" is the basis of most of the recourse and litigation procedures, because the patient feels hit, damaged and above all ignored as a person. The failure of the recognition of the patient's emotions and feelings related to the (eventual) damage causes feelings of anger and a possible aggression to the healthcare professional. The communication procedures that we are discussing can represent an important barrier and help to temper these reactions and help the patient to deal with the problem with the help of his doctor. This certainly entails emotional costs, the need to dedicate time, more time to the patient after a medical error, answering his questions and clarifying any points that may emerge.

A further important aspect is to distinguish what is said, that is, the verbal communication, and how something is said, that is, the non-verbal communication. Since through communication therapeutic relationships are structured, in which therapy procedures are explained and implemented and in which compliance and adherence to treatments are expected, it is essential that in his professional communication, the healthcare professional is aware that there is a verbal level, consisting of the content, that is, the choice of precise words and sentences and a non-verbal level, consisting of the tone of the voice, the mimicry, the look, the smile/friendliness, the touch, the proximity/distance from the patient and the gestures that accompany the communication. Non-verbal communication "comments" on verbal communication can reinforce or weaken it, and it is appropriate that a healthcare professional has done self-observing trial in order to know the way he/she talks, moves, etc. and learn how to control the non-verbal aspects of the communication.

Case Vignette 6

MB is about 60 years old and is accompanied to the emergency room. The patient screams, is agitated and protests loudly. MB was taken to hospital after being blocked by the Vatican police because he absolutely wanted to meet the Pope and also convene the President of the United States. The three of them, he says, could with his powers have ended all wars in the world. The Vatican police did not let him in but the patient insisted repeatedly, until he was angry at the refusal and his explanations and hit them because they hindered him in his great universal mission. While he is waiting for the psychiatrist (called urgently), he speaks loudly with all the nurses and says that he has a mission; they are treating him mad, but they don't understand that he is a genius. The psychiatrist arrives, asks information about the patient, enters the room and introduces himself and says to him: "They told me that you felt engaged in an important mission and you could not speak to the Pope. You felt hindered … that's why did you feel so angry?"

"Very angry? Very angry! And I am also very worried about all the people who die in the world and only I can save them!" The psychiatrist says: "I understand, you feel you have a very important mission but let's talk about it better together, tell me how your idea was born. I also see you very tense and nervous, maybe you may need something that makes you feel a little calmer, with all this tension you may have high blood pressure problems". The patient replies: "Yes, actually I have high blood pressure problems, maybe it's better that I take something". The patient sits in front of the psychiatrist and starts talking.

Thanks to the initial intervention of the psychiatrist, through empathic communication, the doctor builds a bridge between him and the patient, who at the end of the interview accepts voluntary hospitalization.

Case Vignette 5

AC is 30 years old, suffering from severe obsessive-compulsive disorder for many years now. The patient has responded poorly to normal anti-obsessive drug therapy. The obsessions are so intense that he says that often he cannot even finish a speech without going into details. AC tells that he went to two different psychiatrists and a psychotherapist, and after a few minutes that he spoke, they told him that it was obsessive-compulsive disorder, stopping him, and that he had to heal himself, suggesting him to take anti-obsessive drugs, or psychotherapy. The patient had tried to better explain his disorder, but the therapists were of few words and said to him: Yes, of course, it is only obsessive-compulsive disorder!

AC goes to a young psychotherapist, who, after listening to him carefully and letting him speak, said to him: "Of course, it must be really terrible to have your head so invaded by obsessions. I think you are suffering a lot". The patient replies: "Yes, really a lot! And I don't know how to do it. I try to stop them but I can't, I'm desperate because they keep coming and sometimes, I even think I will end my life just to get rid of it".

The therapist says: "I guess you are also very tired and exhausted from the efforts you make and maybe even a little disappointed and angry because you can't. But it's not your fault, it's the obsessions, just the obsessions that are like that".

The patient says, "You finally understood me! You are the first person to understand how bad I am".

This is a good example of emphatic communication, in which the patient feels that his emotions and mental state are recognized, and this is the best way to start a strong therapeutic alliance and try to really help the patient to feel better and work together on his mental disease.

The common fields of application of empathic communication basically involve all those contexts in which a healthcare professional-patient relationship is involved. It represents the first phase of communication with the patient by generating a simple opening, bridging the other and preparing, in the case of the END method, the subsequent phases of normalization and de-escalation. These last two phases could also be used alone, but in clinical experience, they can follow with greater power after building the "empathic bridge". Empathic communication has a cost for the clinician because if in several cases it is easy to represent the mental state of the other and tune in to it, in some cases it can be very difficult and constitute a considerable effort. In these cases, which occur mainly with some patients at the beginning of the training of residents in psychiatry and psychotherapy, careful supervision is necessary. Over time, the student will acquire the ability of a professional communication valid in most cases, also because he will have greatly increased his knowledge of the range of human emotions in critical and different psychopathological situations. For this reason, it's essential to train about "Erlebnis", that is, the subjective psychic experience composed of patients' thoughts and emotions, as the patient feels and lives the individual clinical conditions, like in depression, schizophrenia, anxiety, borderline, narcissistic personality disorders, etc.

So, the most common fields of application are mainly in psychiatry with difficult patients: the angry patient with probable aggressive behaviour; the patient with severe anxiety, such as in panic attack disorder; or the patient with psychomotor agitation; in states of psychotic fear, as happens in schizophrenic states; severe states of demoralization or depression, such as in major or melancholic depression; and delusional states in manic episodes. Beyond these conditions, it can be useful with oppositional patients, who refuse therapies or treatments, or in the management of patients at risk of suicide and in patients with somatization and somatoforms disorders. Empathic communication encounters difficulties in states of acute intoxication by substances and in organic brain disorders such as dementias and in case of mental retardation.

Its common and very valid application is in the psychotherapy setting, particularly in establishing the therapeutic alliance in the early stages. However, it can also be useful in the advanced stages of psychotherapy, to represent possible mental states of the other to be explored and allow further insights. It should be remembered that empathic communication, as it is meant here and for these purposes, must never include judgements and comparisons.

Another important field of application is in general medicine and in particular in oncology.

In oncology, empathy is one of the basic skills of the SPIKES method (setting, perception, invitation for information, knowledge, empathy, summarize and strategize), a skill-based approach proposed by Walter Baile et al. for the communication with cancer patients when giving bad news; discussing treatment choices, after relapses and failure of treatments; and introducing second- or third-line cancer treatments and genetic testing [67, 68].

Another field of application was that of teaching empathic communication in children, to prevent aggressive behaviour towards others.

Pioneer of this clinical research line in children was Norma Feshbach with her training conducted on elementary school students and is still a milestone [69].

A final field of application is that of training psychology, psychiatry and psychotherapy students, who are trained to infer patients' thoughts and emotions, as a fundamental base of their clinical work. In this context, Carl Rogers played a seminal and historical role [70], with further contributions, including Barone et al. [71], Ruesch [72] and Hammond DC and Smith VG [73].

3.5   Is Empathy a Skill for Everyone?

A recent study conducted in Canada on 775 psychotherapists of different orientations found that there are marked differences regarding empathic abilities, with 4 different profiles [74].

The first, 23% of psychotherapists have below average characteristics with poor performance of emotional resonance towards patients and in the cognitive ability to take the other's point of view, more oriented on their negative emotional reactions to the appearance of the other's distress; the second group, of 26% of the clinicians, has empathic levels above average, tending to immerse themselves in the emotional experiences of others, oriented to guess the moods of the other; the third and largest group, 38% of clinicians reflect average empathy, with adequate levels of emotional involvement and occasional experiences of distress during the sessions. There is a fourth profile, with the highest levels of empathic style, 13%, of a rational type and capable of having an intellectual understanding of the patients' perspective, with high ability to regulate interpersonal relationships.

The authors conclude: "The question of how to handle clinicians who appear empathically unfit is an important and thorny issue for the field to consider".

Our hope is that this chapter, and in general a manual like this one, can be helpful to acquire this skill or to better improve empathic communication and subsequently normalization and de-escalation. In our experience of training students and residents, as well as health personnel who participated in the courses on the END method, there is a very promising acquisition of skills, with a relapse referred to after some time in their professional practice (Table 3.4).

The acquisition of empathic skills is possible, and even for those with a low level, appropriate training can help improve this skill. As mentioned above, empathic communication is the first and fundamental step to build a relationship with the patient and allow you to manage difficult situations. Empathic communication skills must be continuously trained. It supports not only the first meeting or the individual emergency situation but also the entire therapeutic path. Based on our experience, some subjects benefit a lot while others less.

One of the risks, a negative effect that we have noticed in some cases, is the acquisition of a "mechanical" empathic ability, or the automatic reproduction of formulas or sentences with an empathic but insincere frame.

Empathic communication cannot be simulated. Another aspect that we have revealed is that it requires preparedness and an attitude with which the healthcare professional comes into contact with the patient. An attitude is needed that sees empathic communication as a professional skill: as you wear the lab coat before making a visit, so you wear a mental state before communicating empathically.

This clearly has a cost in terms of fatigue for the healthcare professional; fatigue is a limit to the ability to be empathetic. We have observed in our experience that the health professional at the beginning of the shift is much more ready and capable of empathetic communication than at the end of the shift, or if he had a very difficult and tiring day. Empathic ability can also be compromised by a conflicting work environment or atmosphere or by a high rate of very aggressive or substance-using patients.

Table 3.4 The table shows the results of an anonymous questionnaire administered following a course on END communication

	Before the END course		After the END course	
	Very low/low Modest	Good/very good	Very low/low Modest	Good/very good
My ability to organize a therapeutic response with very aggressive and difficult patients is currently	64%	36%	18%	82%
My ability to verbally respond to criticism from an angry patient is currently	41%	59%	18%	82%
My knowledge to reduce the risk of escalation and of the uncontrolled increase of emotions of a patient in critical situations are	64%	41%	14%	86%
My knowledge to organize a facility where to welcome patients in psychiatric emergency situations and to establish some management procedures is currently	77%	23%	18%	82%
My ability to answer to a scared patient is currently	32%	68%	5%	95%
My current preparation for using specific phrases and ways to make a patient feel that I understand how he feels is	50%	50%	5%	95%
My ability to negotiate therapeutic goals using specific communication techniques is currently	55%	45%	9%	91%
My ability to communicate to a patient that the experience he is experiencing has also happened to others and that it can therefore be overcome is currently	41%	59%	9%	91%
My ability to respond to a patient in an acute delusional state without drugs—or waiting to start specific drug therapy—is currently	59%	41%	9%	91%
My ability to communicate in an emergency has recently improved	59%	41%	0%	100%

It can also be compromised by personal factors of the healthcare professional, such as phases of life with high intimate stress (loss of a loved one, divorce, a child's illness, serious personal illness, etc.).

It would be useful to have regular group supervision that allows to recognize the difficulties and discuss them and be helped to face the work setting. Therefore, an empathic communication training, and more generally on the END method, does its best within a good work organization, with a leader who recognizes and promotes it.

Unfortunately, in normal clinical experience, not only of a psychiatric/psychological type but also of various specialized disciplines, there is today a great diversity of empathic behaviours, with clinicians who naturally know how to stay close to the patient, and others, who, although in good faith, believe they act well, with harsh and sometimes offensive communications and with little or no attention to the other's mental state or to the patient's emotions.

Case Vignette 7

A.C., a 70-year-old woman, with a severe obsessive-compulsive disorder and an anxious state pervading her daily life, goes accompanied by her psychotherapist to the routine outpatient visit to keep under control a blood disease she has already had for many years, but from the last analyses, the values have risen and have reached borderline values. The patient asks to be accompanied by her psychotherapist precisely because she is afraid of feeling bad from anxiety during the visit, but above all she is terribly frightened by the response of the attending physician, because the blood disease can turn into a cancer. As soon as the patient enters the doctor's room, she is verbally attacked by the doctor: "Here, as usual, you are not accompanied by a family member. I wonder what kind of mother you must have been for never having seen any of your three daughters in all these years". The patient remains motionless, petrified and terrified. The doctor adds: "Well I see that you brought the 'psychological support'. At least so maybe you can stay calmer".

The doctor explains the difficult situation of the blood values of A.C.; the only thing to do is to wait and observe how the disease develops. "Now, you have to react and stay calm, don't stress yourself with all your obsessions and anxiety. It's important that you react and stay calm, but I know you since a lot of years and I'm not sure con can do this … don't stress yourself with stupid things! It's important for your health!"

In this specific case, the communicative style of the doctor is very hard, even if he does it for the good of the patient. The doctor does not understand the emotional state of the patient, and with his harsh tones and words, he tries to encourage the patient to react, but not recognizing her mental state; the doctor worsens the patient's already emotionally serious condition.

We believe that these are not the faults of the poorly empathetic healthcare professional but often have different underlying reasons: the first reason is the defence from the anguish that serious patients arouse in the healthcare professional; the second reason is the identification with an authoritarian model, perhaps learned by a teacher, who appears as a guide in difficult clinical situations and tries to push the patient to a (positive) reaction; and the third reason, perhaps the simplest of all, is that so far most clinicians and health professionals have not been trained in this regard; therefore, they do not recognize the problem and are not aware of the other's mental state and the consequences that this lack has on the patient.

3.6   Summary

Empathy has many definitions; after a brief historical review, in this chapter empathic communication is defined as the ability to recognize the mood of the other and use specific methods to return it to the person. It is vitally important to understand and make others understand that we understand how and what the other one feels, because it is only in this way that we can build a communication bridge between us and the other one and be able to start communication.

In our method, empathic communication is the first step in dealing with normalizing communication and de-escalation. Understood in this sense, empathic communication is simple; it can be very short, even just two or three sentences, but it implies a "know-how" and a particular preparation and professional attitude, not always easy to implement.

As specified several times during this chapter, it is important to know how to do and what to do, having in mind an action plan before starting the empathic communication. In a nutshell, it is important to be prepared and trained for this type of communication.

Several examples of "good" but not empathic communication and "bad" and empathic communication are provided throughout the chapter. The examples concern emergency situations in psychiatry and acute cases, as well as some examples of general and specialistic medicine. Learning the use of empathic communication, and in general the whole END method, can often make the difference.

In our perspective, empathic communication is seen as part of prosocial ethological behaviour with specific dedicated brain circuits (circuits of empathy); consequently, the clinician "speaks" to these circuits and creates an engagement with the patient, working through the words with the brain circuits involved. Particular attention is also given to non-verbal communication aspects (tone of voice, body posture, facial expression, etc.), which are also heavily involved in the empathic communication process.

We hope that the presentation of the empathic communication, but more generally of the END method, will help clinicians to improve their work and, in this way, to help their patients more effectively.

References

1. Pigman GW. Freud and the history of empathy. Int J Psychoanal. 1995;76(Pt 2):237–56.
2. R. Vischer, Über das optische Formgefühl, 1873
3. Lipps T. Ästhetik. Psychologie des Schönen und der Kunst. Hamburg, Leipzig: Voss; 1903/1906.
4. Freud S. Der Witz und seine Beziehung zum Umbewussten. Leipzig, Wien: Franz Deuticke; 1905.
5. Feshbach N. Parental empathy and child adjustment – maladjustment. In: Eisenberg N, Strayer J, editors. Empathy and its development. Cambridge: Cambridge University Press; 1987.
6. Blair RJR. Responding to emotion of others: dissociating forms of empathy trough the study of typical and psychiatric populations. Conscious Cogn. 2005;14:698–718.

7. Williams B, Beovich B. Psychometric properties of the Jefferson Scale of Empathy: a COSMIN systematic review protocol. Syst Rev. 2019;8(1):319.
8. Eisenberg N, Miller P. Empathy and prosocial behaviour. Psychol Bull. 1987;101:91–119.
9. Farrow TFD. Neuroimaging of empathy. In: Farrow T, Woodruff P, editors. Empathy in mental illness. Cambridge: Cambridge University Press; 2007.
10. Heyes C. Empathy is not in our genes. Neurosci Biobehav Rev. 2018;95:499–507.
11. Völlm BA, Taylor AN, Richardson P, Corcoran R, Stirling J, McKie S, Deakin JF, Elliott R. Neuronal correlates of theory of mind and empathy: a functional magnetic resonance imaging study in a nonverbal task. Neuroimage. 2006;29(1):90–8.
12. Brothers L. A biological perspective on empathy. Am J Psychiatry. 1989;146:10.
13. Dunbar RIM. The social brain hypothesis. Evol Anthropol. 1998;6:178.
14. Dunbar RIM. The social brain hypothesis and its implications for social evolution. Ann Hum Biol. 2009;36:562.
15. Frith CD. The social brain? Philos Trans R Soc B. 2007;362:671.
16. Adolphs R. The social brain: neural basis of social knowledge. Annu Rev Psychol. 2009;60:693.
17. Blair RJR. The amygdala and ventromedial prefrontal cortex: functional contributions and dysfunction in psychopathy. Philos Trans R Soc B. 2008;363:2557.
18. Blair RJR. Neurobiological basis of psychopathy. Br J Psychiatry. 2003;182:5.
19. Marsh AA, Finger EC, Fowler KA, Adalio CJ, Jurkowitz TN, Schechter JC, Pine DS, Decety J, Blair RJR. Empathic responsiveness in amygdala and anterior cingulate cortex in youths with psychopathic traits. J Child Psychol Psychiatry. 2013;54:900.
20. Blair RJR. Traits of empathy and anger: implications for psychopathy and other disorders associated with aggression. Philos Trans R Soc B. 2018;373:20170155.
21. Lee KH, Farrows TFD, Spence SA, Woodruff PWR. Social cognition, brain networks and schizophrenia. Psychol Med. 2004;34:391.
22. Hobson PR. Empathy and autism. In: Empathy in mental illness. Cambridge: Cambridge University Press; 2007.
23. Lombardo M, Chakrabarti B, Bullmore E, Sadek SA, Pasco G, Wheelwright SJ, Suckling J, M. A. Consortium, Baron-Cohen S. Atypical neural self-representation in autism. Brain. 2010;133:611.
24. Harlow JM. Recovery from the passage of an iron bar through the head. Waltham, MA: Massachusetts Medical Society; 1868.
25. Shamay-Tsoory SG, Tomer R, Berger B, Aharon-Peretz J. Characterization of empathy deficits following prefrontal brain damage: the role of the right ventromedial prefrontal cortex. J Cogn Neurosci. 2003;15:324.
26. Batson CD. These things called empathy: eight related but distinct phenomena. In: The social neuroscience of empathy. Cambridge, MA: MIT Press; 2009.
27. Smith A. Cognitive empathy and emotional empathy in human behavior and evolution. Psychol Rec. 2006;56:3.
28. Shamay-Tsoory SG, Aharon-Peretz J, Perry D. Two systems for empathy: a double dissociation between emotional and cognitive empathy in inferior frontal gyrus versus ventromedial prefrontal lesions. Brain. 2009;132:617.
29. Baroh-Cohen S. Autism: the empathizing–systemizing (E-S) theory. Ann N Y Acad Sci. 2009;1156:68.
30. Premack D, Woodruff G. Does the chimpanzee have a theory of mind? Behav Brain Sci. 1978;1:515.
31. Wimmer H, Perner J. Beliefs about beliefs: representation and constraircing function of wrong beliefs in young children's understanding of deception. Cognition. 1983;13:103.
32. Baron-Cohen S, Leslie A, Frith U. Does the autistic child have a theory of mind? Cognition. 1985;21:37.
33. Happé FGE. An advanced test of theory of mind: understanding of story characters' thoughts and feelings by able autistic, mentally handicapped, and normal children and adults. J Autism Dev Disord. 1994;24:129.

34. Baron-Cohen S, Wheelwright S, Joliffe T. Is there a "language of the eyes"? Evidence from normal adults, and adults with autism or Asperger Syndrome. Vis Cogn. 1997;4:311.
35. Decety J. Empathy in medicine: what it is, and how much we really need it. Am J Med. 2020;133:561.
36. Blair J, Sellars C, Strickland I, Clark F, Williams A, Smith M, Jones L. Theory of mind in the psychopath. J Foren Psychiatry. 1996;7:15.
37. Richell RA, Mitchell DGV, Newman C, Leonard A, Baron-Cohen S, Blair RJR. Theory of mind and psychopathy: can psychopathic individuals read the 'language of the eyes'? Neuropsychologia. 2003;41:563.
38. Shamay-Tsoory SG, Harari H, Aharon-Peretz J, Levkovitz Y. The role of the orbitofrontal cortex in affective theory of mind deficits in criminal offenders with psychopathic tendencies. Cortex. 2010;46:668.
39. Lehmann A, Bahçesular K, Brockmann EM, Biederbick S, Dziobek I, Gallinat J, Montag C. Subjective experience of emotions and emotional empathy in paranoid schizophrenia. Psychiatry Res. 2014;220:825.
40. Berger P, Bitsch F, Jakobi B, Nagels A, Straube B, Falkenberg I. Cognitive and emotional empathy in patients with schizophrenia spectrum disorders: a replication and extension study. Psychiatry Res. 2019;276:56.
41. Tholen MG, Trautwein F-M, Böckler A. Functional magnetic resonance imaging (fMRI) item analysis of empathy and theory of mind. Hum Brain Mapp. 2020;41:2611.
42. Bzdok D, Schilbach L, Vogeley K, Schneider L, Laird AR, Langner R, Eickhoff SB. Parsing the neural correlates of moral cognition: ALE meta-analysis on morality, theory of mind, and empathy. Brain Struct Funct. 2012;217:783.
43. Schurz M, Radua J, Aichhorn M, Richlan F, Perner J. Fractionating theory of mind: a meta-analysis of functional brain imaging studies. Neurosci Biobehav Rev. 2014;42:9.
44. Eres R, Decety J, Louis WR, Molenberghs P. Individual differences in local gray matter density are associated with differences in affective and cognitive empathy. Neuroimage. 2015;117:305.
45. Kanske P, Böckler A, Trautwein F-M, Singer T. Dissecting the social brain: introducing the EmpaToM to reveal distinct neural networks and brain – behavior relations for empathy and theory of mind. Neuroimage. 2015;122:6.
46. de Waal FBM, Preston SD. Mammalian empathy: behavioural manifestations and neural basis. Nat Rev Neurosci. 2017;18:498.
47. Rizzolati G, Caruana F. Some considerations on de Waal and Preston review. Nat Rev Neurosci. 2017;18:769.
48. Gallese V, Keysers C, Rizzolati G. A unifying view of the basis of social cognition. Trends Cogn Sci. 2004;8:396.
49. Rizzolatti G, Fabbri-Destro M, Cattaneo L. Mirror neurons and their clinical relevance. Nat Clin Pract Neurol. 2009;5:24.
50. Rizzolatti G, Fogassi L, Gallese V. Neurophysiological mechanisms underlying the understanding and imitation of action. Nat Rev Neurosci. 2001;2:661.
51. Rizzolati G, Craighero L. The mirror-neuron system. Annu Rev Neurosci. 2004;27:169.
52. Iacoboni M, Molnar-Szakacs M, Gallese V, Buccino G, Mazziotta JC. Grasping the intentions of others with one's own mirror neuron system. PLoS Biol. 2005;3:e79.
53. Gallese V. The roots of empathy: the shared manifold hypothesis and the neural basis of intersubjectivity. Psychopathology. 2003;36:171.
54. Preston SD, de Wall FBM. Empathy: its ultimate and proximate bases. Behav Brain Sci. 2002;25:1.
55. Marsh AA, Yu H, Pine DS, Blair RJR. Oxytocin improves specific recognition of positive facial expressions. Psychopharmacology (Berl). 2010;209:225.
56. Hurlemann R, Patin A, Onur OA, Coehn MX, Baumgartner T, Metzler S, Dziobek I, Gallinat J, Wagner M, Maier W, Kendrik K. Oxytocin enhances amygdala-dependent, socially reinforced learning and emotional empathy in humans. J Neurosci. 2010;30:4999.
57. Fragkaki I, Cima M. The effect of oxytocin administration on empathy and emotion recognition in residential youth: a randomized, within-subjects trial. Horm Behav. 2019;114:104561.

58. Domes G, Ower N, von Dawans B, Spengler FB, Dziobek I, Bohus M, Matthies S, Philipsen A, Heinrichs M. Effects of intranasal oxytocin administration on empathy and approach motivation in women with borderline personality disorder: a randomized controlled trial. Transl Psychiatry. 2019;9:328.
59. Halverson T, Jarskog LF, Pedersen C, Penn D. Effects of oxytocin on empathy, introspective accuracy, and social symptoms in schizophrenia: a 12-week twice-daily randomized controlled trial. Schizophr Res. 2019;204:178.
60. Palgi S, Klein E, Shamay-Tsoory S. The role of oxytocin in empathy in PTSD. Psychol Trauma Theory Res Pract Policy. 2017;9:70.
61. Geng Y, Zhao W, Zhou F, Ma X, Yao S, Hurlemann R, Becker B, Kendrick KM. Oxytocin enhancement of emotional empathy: generalization across cultures and effects on amygdala activity. Front Neurosci. 2018;12:512.
62. de Vignemont F, Singer T. The empathic brain: how, when and why? Trends Cogn Sci. 2006;10:435.
63. Bernhardt BC, Singer T. The neural basis of empathy. Annu Rev Neurosci. 2012;35:1.
64. Singer T, Lamm C. The social neuroscience of empathy. Ann N Y Acad Sci. 2009;1156:81.
65. Jimenez KCB, Abdelgabar A, De Angelis L, McKay L, Keysers C, Gazzola V. Changes in brain activity following the voluntary control of empathy. Neuroimage. 2020;216:116529.
66. Santamaría-García H, Baez S, García AM, Flichtentrei D, Prats M, Mastandueno R, Sigman M, Matallana D, Cetkovich M, Ibanez A. Empathy for others' suffering and its mediators in mental health professionals. Sci Rep. 2017;7:6391.
67. Baile WF. Giving bad news. Oncologist. 2015;20(8):852–3.
68. I*CARE. Interpersonal communication and relationship enhancement. Basic principles. http://www.mdanderson.org/education-and-research/resources-for-professionals/professional-educational-resources/i-care/complete-library-of-communication-videos/basic-principles.html.
69. Feshbach N. Empathy, empathy training and the regulation of aggression in elementary school children. In: Kaplan RM, Konecni VJ, Novaco RW, editors. Aggression in children and youth. The Hague; Boston, MA; Lancaster: Martinus Nijhoff Publishers; 1984.
70. Rogers CR. Counselling and psychotherapy. New York, NY: Houghton Muffin; 1970.
71. Ruesch J, Hammond DC, Barone DF, Hutchings PS, Kimmel HJ, Traub HL, Cooper JT, Marshall CM. Increasing empathic accuracy through practice and feedback in a clinical interviewing course. J Soc Clin Psychol. 2005;24(2):156–71.
72. Ruesch J. Therapeutic communication. New York, NY: Norton; 1973.
73. Hammond DC, Hepworth DH, Smith VG. Improving therapeutic communication. San Francisco, CA: Jossey-Bass; 1979.
74. Laverdière O, Kealy D, Ogrodniczuk JS, Descôteaux J. Got empathy? A latent profile analysis of psychotherapists' empathic abilities. Psychother Psychosom. 2019;88(1):41–2.

The End Method: Normalization

4

Francesco Saverio Bersani and Roberto Delle Chiaie

4.1 Introduction to the Concept

Normalization has a relevant role within the END (empathy, normalization, de-escalation) method, conceptualized to facilitate the communication with patients with severe mental diseases (SMDs) during the critical periods of the course of their illnesses as well as during emerging emotional crisis. Normalization has been defined in relation to mental diseases by Kingdon and Turkington as *"the process by which thoughts, behaviors, moods and experiences are compared and understood in terms of similar thoughts, behaviors, moods and experiences attributed to other individuals who are not diagnosed as ill"* [1] and by Dudley et al. as *"a process that emphasises that the experiences a person finds upsetting exist within the range of normal functioning and can be experienced in the absence of distress, or disability"* [2].

Normalization is a technique traditionally used within the context of cognitive behavioural therapy (CBT) [2, 3]. It is based on the idea that, consistently with the pioneering work of Lazarus and Folkman on the topic [4], the different ways psychopathological or environmental events are viewed and appraised by an individual can differently modulate emotions, behaviours, and underlying psychobiological responses [2, 3].

The implementation of a normalization approach for patients with psychiatric disorders usually implies the integrated use of a range of strategies connected to CBT, including the ABC model, the identification of reasoning errors and automatic thoughts, the use of analogies, the cognitive restructuration, and the evaluation of records. Group settings may be especially useful: being in a group can represent an important normalizing process for patients as within the group they can realize and understand that their symptoms and problems are similarly experienced by other

F. S. Bersani (✉) · R. Delle Chiaie
Department of Human Neurosciences, Sapienza University of Rome, Rome, Italy
e-mail: francescosaverio.bersani@uniroma1.it; r.dellechiaie@centrokahlbaum.it

© Springer Nature Switzerland AG 2021
M. Biondi et al. (eds.), *Empathy, Normalization and De-escalation*,
https://doi.org/10.1007/978-3-030-65106-0_4

people, thus receiving a "you are not alone" encouraging message [5]. Personal disclosures in which clinicians provide information on personal experiences related to their own past psychological disturbances can in some cases facilitate the organization of good therapeutic relationships and can support patients in feeling their conditions as common [2, 3, 6].

Several clinical objectives can be addressed by means of a normalization process, among which decatastrophizing the meaning of psychopathological events for the individual, improving the feeling of control over the symptoms, reducing anxiety, ameliorating engagement and adherence to treatment, reducing maladaptive emotional reactions, and increasing the understanding of (1) psychopathological phenomena, (2) the effects on individuals of stigma and discrimination, and (3) the effects of psychosocial stressors in exacerbating psychiatric symptoms.

To the best of our knowledge, there are no studies aimed at exploring the biological underpinnings of normalization interventions; however, robust evidence suggests that CBT can influence a range of physiological and molecular pathways [7]. It has been suggested that (1) normalizing interventions contribute to change the emotional state of patients, potentially leading individuals who feel fear, rage, or terror to experience increased levels of calm and tranquillity, and (2) that this may occur through the modulation of pathways related to fear perception (mainly involving the prefrontal cortex, thalamus, amygdala, hypothalamus, and locus coeruleus) [8].

Certain psychological concepts, such as psychoeducation, mental health stigmatization, stress-related psychiatric symptoms, decatastrophization, symptom-based continuum perspective, treatment adherence, and minimization, are tightly related to normalization, and their understanding is thus an integral part of normalization approaches.

Psychoeducation has been defined by Bauml et al. as a *"behavioural therapeutic concept consisting of 4 elements: briefing the patients about their illness, problem solving training, communication training, and self-assertiveness training"* [9]. The use of psychoeducation in SMDs has been receiving increasing attention, and robust evidence supports its clinical usefulness [9–11]. At the biological level, our research group recently showed that group psychoeducation can have a role in ameliorating neuroendocrine physiology in patients with bipolar disorder (BD) under pharmacological maintenance treatment contributing to normalize cortisol awakening response [12, 13]. As among the objectives of normalization approaches there are the improvement of patients' understanding of psychopathological phenomena and the reduction of maladaptive emotional reactions such as anxiety, concern of being anxious, demoralization, and dissatisfaction of feeling melancholic, it is important that psychoeducation is included and integrated in the framework of such interventions. Psychoeducational approaches such as providing patients handouts, clarifications, and worksheets related to their disturbances may be helpful within normalization processes.

Mental health stigmatization has been defined by Hayward and Bright as *"the negative effects of a label placed on any group, such as a racial or religious minority, or, in this case, those who have been diagnosed as mentally ill"* [14], as, for example, *"if a person threatens his neighbours he will not be well thought of, but many argue that he will incur an additional negative opinion from those neighbours if they believe that his behaviour is caused by mental illness*" [14]. Evidence suggests that perceived stigma and perceived discrimination can negatively influence treatment outcomes for patients with psychiatric disorders as they contribute to reduce access to care and they contribute to promote wrong knowledge about the features and treatability of the disorders [15]. Normalizing interventions can help patients in having a more correct and "normalized" view of their own condition, symptoms, and expectations, thus reducing the impact of the society-induced stigma on their perception of themselves as individuals with a psychiatric disorder [1, 16]. Further, an additional goal to achieve during the normalization interventions is to help patients to realize that they are not alone in experiencing their condition and this can possibly support them in reducing their perceived stigma, increasing their self-esteem, and improving their coping skills.

The concept of stress-related psychiatric symptoms refers to the evidence that there are certain physiological or psychosocial conditions that may induce or exacerbate psychiatric symptoms and that, subsequently, experiencing psychiatric symptoms does not necessarily mean being affected by a chronic disabling condition, but rather it can be the transient consequence of certain acute circumstances [17]. The stress-vulnerability model, in fact, implies that individuals can have a predisposition towards the development of mental disorders but that psychiatric symptoms including depressive, manic, and psychotic episodes fully manifest in response to environmental/psychosocial stressors [17]. Normalization approaches may subsequently assist patients in accepting the idea that virtually everybody can experience high levels of painful emotional distress and in identifying those recurrent circumstances which can trigger the worsening of their symptoms [1, 2]. As suggested by Kingdon and Turkington, in relation to stress-related psychiatric symptoms, "*normalization seems to assist by promoting self-esteem, reducing the feeling of estrangement from others, and appropriately reattributing experiences that may seem externally generated to internal causes*" [1].

Catastrophic thinking has been described as a cognitive distortion contributing to the onset and worsening of psychopathological phenomena and representing an indicator of poor health and mental health outcomes [18]. Patients with psychiatric disorders can catastrophize the signs and symptoms related to their own diseases as well as physiological unrelated sensations; helping the patients to decatastrophize the beliefs on their conditions is considered an important element for the success of normalization interventions [1, 16].

It has been reported that all individuals can experience some level of psychopathological symptoms in diverse occasions during life and that subsequently a symptom-based continuum perspective can more closely resemble the nature of psychiatric disturbances than a categorical approach [19, 20]. Research on such view of psychopathology has recently been stimulated by the Research Domain Criteria [21]. Subsequently, a normalizing intervention can support patients in avoiding to see their own condition as a yes/no healthy/sick dichotomous state and rather in considering the degree of psychological functioning as a continuum which everybody make efforts to manage and control.

Most of the times, treatment adherence of patients with severe psychiatric diseases is low, with studies suggesting that interventions aimed at improving individual functioning level or the degree of social support can play an ameliorating role [22]. Adherence to treatment often depends on the relationship between the prescribing physician and the patient. Lencer et al. suggested that normalization can represent a valuable option during adherence assessment or intervention [23]; the authors suggested, among the other things, that framing discussion on non-adherence problems in terms of desired outcomes, and not of obedience, keeping the discussion on medication adherence as positive or enjoyable, conveying curiosity in a non-judgemental fashion, addressing the lack of insight, avoiding the use of fear communication, taking harm reduction approaches, and understanding patient's perspective on medication efficacy, are psychological strategies related to normalization which can support the therapist in increasing patients' adherence to treatment [23].

As pointed out by Dudley et al., *"care should be taken that normalisation is not used in the extreme, which may be perceived to minimize the problem"* [2]. Efforts to normalize a symptom, in fact, may be perceived by patients as minimizations of the problem, with this potentially leading to the worsening of therapeutic relationship.

4.2 Normalization in the Clinical Management of Severe Mental Disorders and other Medical Conditions

Schizophrenia (SCZ), BD, and major depressive disorder (MDD) are often referred to as SMDs, and normalizing interventions have been used in such conditions.

CBT has been extensively studied for treatment of MDD, with studies indicating the combination of CBT and antidepressants as an effective therapeutic option for such condition [24, 25]. As reported by Wright et al., normalizing messages in relation to severe depression can be focused on the facts that depression is an extremely common condition and it can be related to other medical illnesses, that there are research programs being conducted in order to elucidate the aetiology and pathophysiology of depression, and that there is robust evidence suggesting good clinical response to antidepressants and to psychotherapy [26]. "It is not unusual feeling down after an unpleasant experience", "we have seen and succesfully treated several people with problems similar to yours", "many people in your condition would feel like you feel now", "it is normal for you to feel worried, but together we can handle your emotional distress", "a large amount of people may present a severe depressive episode throughout life", are examples of simple but potentially useful and reassuring normalizing statements that health profesionals may say to patients with emotional distress related to depressive symptoms.

In relation to BD, evidence indicating high rates of unmet needs and long-term deficits at the psychological, neurocognitive, and psychosocial level among BD patients in the euthymic phase of the disease, i.e. among those patients who have adequately responded to pharmacotherapy, has stimulated the interest over interventions additional to pharmacotherapy, among which CBT and, subsequently, certain aspects of normalization [24, 26, 27]. Previous findings from our research team suggest that BD patients can show electroencephalographic and neuropsychological anomalies compared to healthy controls even when their mood episodes are remitted, i.e. when they do not show manic/hypomanic or depressive symptoms [28–30], thus supporting the potential importance of identifying additional interventions complementary to pharmacotherapy. Our group recently showed that certain rehabilitative introversions including some aspects of normalization (e.g. psychoeducation, self-monitoring, work for goals) can lead euthymic BD patients to relevant improvements in domains related to cognitive ad social functioning [31]. As suggested by Wright et al., normalization interventions in BD patients can be focused on the self-monitoring of symptoms, supporting the patients in the identification of signs which should not be overinterpreted and signs which should be recognized as potential disease indicators [26]. "It will be hard, but lots of people have faced problems similar to yours, and we will do our best to support you", "people often remain stunned after receiving the same diagnosis you got", "you have faced many critical situations in the past, even this time you will make it", "many successful people have similar disturbances", "don't be afraid to talk to us about the feelings that you experience, even if they may seem not important" are examples of simple but potentially useful and reassuring normalizing statements that health profesionals may say to patients with emotional distress related to BD.

For what concerns SCZ and other psychotic disorders, over the last years, there has been an increasing interest over the use of CBT as a supportive intervention to be integrated with psychopharmacology, and relevant attention has been provided to normalization approaches [1–3, 24, 26, 32, 33]. One of the first studies on the topic was performed by Kingdon and Turkington: the authors used a specific CBT approach with a normalizing rationale in 64 SCZ patients as an adjunct to standard treatment, observing that patients were maintained on low levels of or no medication and required minimal hospitalization [32]. Since then, several further studies have suggested the usefulness of such approach for SCZ individuals as well as for patients with psychotic symptoms in general [24, 34], although a recent meta-analysis suggested that the effect of CBT on functioning at end of trials in patients with psychoses is significant but small [35]. "Under pressure the brain can easily develop delusional thoughts and hallucinations; it is a part of the normal human condition", "we all have a specific stress threshold, above which we can experience unusual thoughts or irrational fears", "many famous people hear (or have heard) voices", "prolonged duration of symptoms and treatment is not exclusively related to psychiatric diseases, but rather it can occur in many common medical conditions", "people may have several side effects when taking these medications, if you will not tolerate them we will find together valid alternatives" are examples of simple but potentially useful and reassuring normalizing statements that health professionals may say to patients with emotional distress related to psychotic disorders.

Wright et al. have recently summarized the modality through which normalization interventions may be targeted on the specific symptom manifestation of SCZ such as hallucinations, delusions, thought disturbances, and negative symptoms [26]; according to the authors, normalization can be focused, among the other things, on helping patients to reduce feelings of loneliness and shame, on providing patients information on how physiological conditions can lead to symptoms, on supporting patients in identifying strategies to control/modulate the intensity of symptoms, thus increasing their sense of empowerment, on developing adaptive coping strategies, and on explaining to patients how mind and body need time to recuperate after severe life events such as acute psychotic episodes [26].

Dudley et al. have described a model in which components such as engagement of patients, organization of a therapeutic alliance, tracing antecedents of psychotic breakdowns, normalization, decatastrophization, education about illness, stress vulnerability models, evidence evaluation, generation of alternative hypotheses, and evaluation of coping strategies are integrated within a form of CBT intervention specifically designed for patients with psychotic disorders [2]. Useful examples in which normalization approaches (mainly based on the discussion of the stress-related model of psychiatric symptoms) have been successfully used in the context of comprehensive interventions for patients with psychotic disorders have been reported by Guidi et al. [36].

Of relevance, it is known that SMDs such as MDD, BD, and SCZ can present with a variety of symptoms which are markedly inter-individually different, i.e. subjects with the same diagnosis can differ in terms of clinical features. As described by Biondi et al. [20, 37], dimensions such as apprehension, fear, sadness, demoralization, anger, aggressiveness, obsessiveness, apathy, impulsivity, reality distortion, thought disorganization, somatization and activation can be present with different degrees of intensity in virtually all the psychiatric disorders; subsequently, it is important that normalization interventions are not driven exclusively by the categorical diagnosis per se, but rather by the individual psychopathological, symptomatic, and cognitive profile of each patient.

It is also important to observe that distressful emotional feelings do not occur exclusively in the context of SMDs, but rather they can be present in patients with somatic diseases who experience anxiety, anger, fear, or demoralization in relation to their health status. Adequate doctor-patient communication can lead to better clinical outcomes and to improved satisfaction of patients, and such form of dialogue has been defined as "*the heart and art of medicine*" [38]. Normalization can in some cases be part of patient-physician communication, and normalizing statements (e.g. "it may be hard to overcome the consequences of such medical condition, but you are not alone in this: other patients are making similar efforts, and we will give you all our support", "it is physiological feeling exhausted after a surgical intervention", "don't be afraid, the majority of people with similar disturbances usually recover quickly") can play a role in reducing reactive emotional distress, thus ameliorating the adhesion of patients to clinical procedures [16].

References

1. Kingdon DG, Turkington D. Psychoeducation and normalization. In: Cognitive therapy of schizophrenia. New York, NY: The Guilford Press; 2005. p. 83–95.
2. Dudley R, et al. Techniques in cognitive behavioural therapy: using normalising in schizophrenia. Tidsskrift for Norsk psykologforening. 2007;44(5):562–72.

3. Dudley R, Turkinton D. Using normalising in cognitive behavioural therapy for schizophrenia. In: Hagen R, et al., editors. CBT for psychosis: a symptom-based approach. London: Routledge; 2011. p. 77–85.
4. Biggs A, Brough P, Drummond S. Lazarus and Folkman's psychological stress and coping theory. In: Cooper CL, Quick JC, editors. The handbook of stress and health: a guide to research and practice. 1st ed. Hoboken, NJ: John Wiley & Sons Ltd; 2017.
5. Finucane A, Mercer SW. An exploratory mixed methods study of the acceptability and effectiveness of mindfulness-based cognitive therapy for patients with active depression and anxiety in primary care. BMC Psychiatry. 2006;6:14.
6. Ziv-Beiman S. Therapist self-disclosure as an integrative intervention. J Psychother Integr. 2013;23(1):59–74.
7. Roffman JL, et al. Neuroimaging and the functional neuroanatomy of psychotherapy. Psychol Med. 2005;35(10):1385–98.
8. Biondi M. Comunicazione medico paziente e mappa di azione. In: Comunicazione con il paziente: il metodo END. Rome: Alpes Italia; 2014. p. 89–102.
9. Bauml J, et al. Psychoeducation: a basic psychotherapeutic intervention for patients with schizophrenia and their families. Schizophr Bull. 2006;32(Suppl 1):S1–9.
10. Tursi MF, et al. Effectiveness of psychoeducation for depression: a systematic review. Aust N Z J Psychiatry. 2013;47(11):1019–31.
11. Colom F. The evolution of psychoeducation for bipolar disorder: from lithium clinics to integrative psychoeducation. World Psychiatry. 2014;13(1):90–2.
12. Delle Chiaie R, et al. Effects of group psychoeducation on stress reactivity neuroendocrine profile in stabilized bipolar patients. A controlled study. Riv Psichiatr. 2019;54(3):120–6.
13. Delle Chiaie R, et al. Group psychoeducation normalizes cortisol awakening response in stabilized bipolar patients under pharmacological maintenance treatment. Psychother Psychosom. 2013;82(4):264–6.
14. Hayward P, Bright JA. Stigma and mental illness: a review and critique. J Ment Health. 1997;6(4):345–54.
15. Henderson C, Evans-Lacko S, Thornicroft G. Mental illness stigma, help seeking, and public health programs. Am J Public Health. 2013;103(5):777–80.
16. Delle Chiaie R. La comunicazione normalizzante. In: Biondi M, editor. Comunicazione con il paziente: il metodo END. Rome: Alpes Italia; 2014. p. 124–39.
17. Goh C, Agius M. The stress-vulnerability model how does stress impact on mental illness at the level of the brain and what are the consequences? Psychiatr Danub. 2010;22(2):198–202.
18. Moore E, et al. Assessing catastrophic thinking associated with debilitating mental health conditions. Disabil Rehabil. 2018;40(3):317–22.
19. Biondi M, Pasquini M. Dimensional psychopharmacology in somatising patients. Adv Psychosom Med. 2015;34:24–35.
20. Biondi M, Pasquini M, Picardi A. Dimensional psychopathology. Cham: Springer International Publishing; 2018.
21. Insel TR. The NIMH Research Domain Criteria (RDoC) Project: precision medicine for psychiatry. Am J Psychiatry. 2014;171(4):395–7.
22. Stentzel U, et al. Predictors of medication adherence among patients with severe psychiatric disorders: findings from the baseline assessment of a randomized controlled trial (Tecla). BMC Psychiatry. 2018;18(1):155.
23. Lencer R, et al. Using CBT to assess to assess and improve adherence. In: When psychopharmacology is not enough. Cambridge: Hogrefe Publishing; 2011. p. 73–7.
24. Thase ME, Kingdon D, Turkington D. The promise of cognitive behavior therapy for treatment of severe mental disorders: a review of recent developments. World Psychiatry. 2014;13(3):244–50.
25. Hofmann SG, et al. The efficacy of cognitive behavioral therapy: a review of meta-analyses. Cogn Ther Res. 2012;36(5):427–40.

26. Wright JH, et al. Normalizing and educating. In: Cognitive-behavior therapy for severe mental illness: an illustrated guide. Washington, DC: American Psychiatric Publishing; 2009. p. 51–74.
27. Chiang KJ, et al. Efficacy of cognitive-behavioral therapy in patients with bipolar disorder: a meta-analysis of randomized controlled trials. PLoS One. 2017;12(5):e0176849.
28. Bernabei L, et al. A preliminary study on hot and cool executive functions in bipolar disorder and on their association with emotion regulation strategies. Riv Psichiatr. 2018;53(6):331–5.
29. Bersani G, et al. Facial expression in patients with bipolar disorder and schizophrenia in response to emotional stimuli: a partially shared cognitive and social deficit of the two disorders. Neuropsychiatr Dis Treat. 2013;9:1137–44.
30. Bersani FS, et al. P300 component in euthymic patients with bipolar disorder type I, bipolar disorder type II and healthy controls: a preliminary event-related potential study. Neuroreport. 2015;26(4):206–10.
31. Bernabei L, et al. Cognitive remediation for the treatment of neuropsychological disturbances in subjects with euthymic bipolar disorder: findings from a controlled study. J Affect Disord. 2020;273:576–85.
32. Kingdon DG, Turkington D. The use of cognitive behavior therapy with a normalizing rationale in schizophrenia. Preliminary report. J Nerv Ment Dis. 1991;179(4):207–11.
33. Lencer R, et al. When psychopharmacology is not enough. Cambridge: Hogrefe Publishing; 2011.
34. Hazell CM, et al. A systematic review and meta-analysis of low intensity CBT for psychosis. Clin Psychol Rev. 2016;45:183–92.
35. Laws KR, et al. Cognitive Behavioural Therapy for schizophrenia - outcomes for functioning, distress and quality of life: a meta-analysis. BMC Psychol. 2018;6(1):32.
36. Guidi A, et al. Le esperienze italiane di trattamento cognitivo-comportamentale dei deliri e delle allucinazioni. In: Fowler D, Garety P, Kuipers E, editors. Terapia cognitivo-comportamentale delle psicosi. Paris: Masson; 1998.
37. Biondi M. L'approccio per dimensioni psicopatologiche. In: Comunicazione con il paziente: il metodo END. Rome: Alpes Italia; 2014. p. 56–88.
38. Ha JF, Longnecker N. Doctor-patient communication: a review. Ochsner J. 2010;10(1):38–43.

De-escalation Techniques in Various Settings

5

Tommaso Accinni, Georgios Papadogiannis, and Luigi Orso

5.1   Introduction

A lot of confusion surrounds the concepts of aggressiveness, agitation, and psychomotor activation due to difficulty in reaching a valid definition of these notions and due to frequent overlapping of their characteristics. However, it is highly important to shed light on this question in order to define appropriate interventions and approaches which would allow to safely and effectively assist people with such behaviors. In this framework, we might consider aggressiveness as a set of behaviors and conducts which are oriented toward harming oneself or others. Aggressiveness can be expressed verbally or behaviorally, and different levels of intention and consciousness may characterize specific conditions and behaviors. More specifically, there is evidence that mental disease represents a risk factor for aggression events, which may happen in different settings such as emergency rooms, hospitals wards, inpatient units, and community and primary care settings [1]. At present it is known that almost one in five patients hospitalized in acute psychiatric wards may commit an act of violence. Risk factors related to violence in psychiatric wards overlap with the ones present among individual patients (male gender, diagnosis of schizophrenia, substance use, and lifetime history of violence) [2]. It is not straightforward to obtain accurate statistics about violence in medical workplace given the difficulty to provide a unique definition. Thirty-five percent to 80% of healthcare personnel, in particular in the context of the emergency department (ED), experienced physical violence at least once, and any one of them experienced verbal violence in their career [3]. Emergency departments are the most vulnerable in regard to violence from patients [4], and part of the reason is the lack of protocols and well-trained operators. Emergency department conditions, patients' critical states, and high-stress environment are other reasons for vulnerability to physical

T. Accinni (✉) · G. Papadogiannis · L. Orso
Department of Human Neuroscience, Policlinico Umberto I of Rome,
Sapienza University of Rome, Rome, Lazio, Italy

© Springer Nature Switzerland AG 2021
M. Biondi et al. (eds.), *Empathy, Normalization and De-escalation*,
https://doi.org/10.1007/978-3-030-65106-0_5

and verbal violence toward healthcare operators [5]. Increasing violence rate in emergency departments has become an increasingly important issue that needs further research.

While conscious of the complexity in considering the relation between violence, aggressive conducts, and mental health, given the risk of prejudice, stigma, and simplified assumptions, clinical evidence suggests that severe mental disorders are a risk factor for violent episodes compared to general population [6, 7]. Moreover, it is well documented that substance use entails a risk increase for violent episodes [8], and the [9] NICE guidelines suggest that substance use is related to violence manifestation, while mental health disorders basically represent a predictive factor, not related to violence in a deterministic way. It appears fundamental to define a set of techniques and guidelines in order to improve prevention and reduce damage risk for patients, healthcare operators, and family members who can often be victims of violence. Rage and anger are interacting conditions situated in an emotional continuum, representing different modes of being. Angry people attempt to overwhelm others, forcing agreement and trying to be heard. Different conditions in terms of lack of social skills, such as mental illness or the effects of drugs and alcohol intoxication, may cause resort to anger which could be considered as a dysfunctional path to communicate feelings and emotions.

Considering that an aggressive episode usually consists of standard subsequent steps, starting from a relatively calm situation and ending in an equally calm condition, an aggression cycle has been described in the scientific literature [10]. The majority of violent episodes can be triggered by specific elements which activate the aggression cycle, even though under certain circumstances may commence spontaneously. More specifically, at baseline people can be considered as quiet and calm, willing to establish interactions, available to dialogue, and able to use refined cognitive resources. In this context, a specific event may represent a trigger element impairing cognitive processes as well as emotional dimension. This event may be threatening or overtly dangerous, leading at first to a sense of frustration and coercion and subsequently to anger. Overtly angry people are irritable, frustrated, verbally aggressive, domineering, and displaying a dismissive, presumptuous, and arrogant attitude; they do not tolerate being contradicted. However, even though in a dysfunctional way, they are trying to communicate to others their feeling and intentions. When anger reaches a higher level of intensity, individuals are less willing or able to negotiate and talk and becoming increasingly aggressive. The progressive escalation is accompanied by an increasing physical activation which worsens the sense of frustration. At this point, an angry person could become enraged, reaching a higher state of activation with decreased inhibitory control resulting in an impairment of the fear of consequences, sense of morality, coherent self-image, or appropriate public image. An enraged person has lost original purpose, becoming unable to communicate thoughts or feelings and aiming to dominate and destroy. The outcome of such conditions may be overt violence with the attempt to hurt, as well as the infliction of fear of imminent physical harm or personal boundaries violation. Potentially dangerous situations originate from extreme emotional disturbances involving vulnerable people with impaired perception and cognition, regardless of the original source of such behavior. In dealing with such complicated situations, diagnosis does not appear crucial in comparison with a potentially dangerous behavior which may represent a risk given its apparent unpredictability. Therefore, conducts and behaviors should be primarily addressed well before categorical diagnosis [13].

5.2   Definition and Concept Evolution

Given the complexity and importance of therapeutic alliance, we may define de-escalation as a process comprising the ability to gradually resolve a potentially violent situation. This process consists of different paths of communication, both verbal and nonverbal, all aimed to set up an alliance based on empathy, comprehension, and non-confrontational dialogue.

Although in recent years several studies have proposed different theoretical models of de-escalation, there is striking lack of evidence about its efficacy in managing aggressiveness and violent episodes. There is need for a structured conceptualization of the concept which would allow to theorize an empirical model in order to guide research and studies. The lack of a structured conceptualization has led to different approaches consisting of non-comparable aspects of the same intervention.

Different studies have sought to provide a conceptual analysis of de-escalation, in order to prompt an evidence-based model of healthcare intervention which would represent a guideline in facing emotional and critical situations at risk for violent conducts. These attempts defined de-escalation as a "collective term for a range of interwoven staff-delivered components comprising communication, self-regulation, assessment, actions, and safety maintenance which aim to extinguish or reduce patient aggression/agitation irrespective of its cause, and improve staff-patient relationships while eliminating or minimizing coercion or restriction."

As stated by NICE guidelines [9], de-escalation is conceived as an attitude based on emotional regulation and procedures oriented toward self-management to avert and prevent aggressive behaviors and violence risk. Furthermore, since the early stage of its theorization, de-escalation has been related to aggressiveness, more specifically to "the assault cycle" involving trigger elements, escalation phase, crisis phase, recovery phase, and depression phase, as described by Kaplan (1983) [14].

De-escalation is conceived as part of the process of managing aggression, and it is considered both as a preventive measure and the most reliable technique to avoid patient aggressiveness' deterioration. Because of that, considering again NICE guidelines, pharmacological rapid tranquilization, physical interventions, and seclusion restraints should be considered only when verbal and nonverbal de-escalation techniques have failed in reducing tension and agitation, leading to the inability to establish a relation. For this reason, it appears clear that de-escalation procedures are not based on common sense and improvisation. Their reliability is built on theorization, procedural techniques, and clinical experience. A complex net of abilities is needed, based on communication and relational skills, aimed to abort the assault cycle and the aggressiveness escalation phase [13]. This background of procedures, which come from theoretical reasoning and clinical experience, not always seems to be feasible, given the resources and staff preparation required. Especially in emergency settings, it is frequently necessary to sedate the patient who will perceive a less traumatic experience compared to restraining procedures, in a first time leaving aside de-escalation procedures [11, 12].

5.3   Neurobiological Correlates

Aggressiveness represents a transnosographic condition involving different psychiatric features. In the present state of knowledge, common neurophysiological underpinnings regarding neurotransmitter pathways and hormonal systems have been described as underlying possible aggressive manifestations in different psychiatric conditions. Therefore, an overarching neurophysiological system involving a common final pathway for aggressive episodes and behavioral dysfunction which could be related to psychopathology should be hypothesized [15].

From an evolutionary point of view, aggression could be conceived as a psychobiological state aimed at defense and protection [16]. When aggressiveness appears related to non-conflictual contexts, without any kind of derivability, and showing no motivation or reason which could explain such a reaction, it represents a dysfunctional condition reflecting specific medical and pathological conditions. Aggression can be externally directed or self-oriented, as observed in many psychiatric disorders or in the frame of drug abuse. As mentioned before, there are several situations which could represent a trigger for aggressive behaviors: aggressiveness may be elicited by provocation and stimulant interactions, appearing in these cases as a reactive state, or it could manifest apparently without any obvious motive.

More specifically, it has been documented that neuropsychological underpinnings of aggressive behavior may overlap with those underlying stress reactions. Moreover, aggressive conducts can be detrimental for individual's health involving neurovegetative, cardiovascular, endocrinological, and immunological reactions. The HPA axis (hypothalamic-pituitary-adrenal axis) is strongly associated with stress reaction, leading to a profound cortisol release [17]. This cascade of events has been observed during aggressive behaviors, being related to the neurobiology underlying violent episodes. We should consider aggressive behavior as an attempt by human beings and animals to cope with stress, supported by activation of stress-induced neurobiological reactions regarding both derivable and pathological aggressiveness. In particular, stress represents a complex system of responses which also may involve detrimental processes and could provoke aggressive conducts. It has been observed that immunological activation intercedes with neuropsychiatric dysfunctions and abnormal behaviors. The pituitary release of the adrenocorticotropic hormone (ACTH) determines the central cortisol secretion [18]. There is evidence that the HPA axis may be associated to aggressive conducts, due to either hyperactivation or inhibition which is related to the negative feedback mechanism of cortisol release [19]. Cortisol release influences the synthesis and the secretion of testosterone, and even more interestingly, it determines behaviors, conducts, and emotional reactions such as anxiety and distress [20]. Furthermore, aggressive conducts may be caused by significant aggressive traits in presence of specific personality characteristics [21]. Hypoarousal-derived aggressiveness has been associated with antisocial personality disorder, involving glucocorticoid hypoactivity; on the other hand, hyperarousal-driven aggressive behaviors may derive from an abnormally hyperactivated glucocorticoid reaction, as it has been observed in the frame of specific neuropsychiatric features such as post-traumatic stress disorder (PTSD) and intermittent explosive disorder [22]. Since the discovery of the neuropeptides, their fundamental role in the regulation of homeostasis, stress-driven events, and motivated behavior has been evidenced [23]. Peripherally synthetized neuropeptides act on brain systems crossing the blood-brain barrier or passing through the perivascular spaces via diffusion, determining in this way a systemic interdependent network. It seems very interesting that specific regions in the brain are surrounded by easily permeable capillaries, representing therefore sensitive regions susceptible to the influence of peripheral peptide hormones such as the median eminence located in close proximity to the ventromedial hypothalamic nucleus which has been associated with the regulation of aggressiveness [24]. Aggressive conducts seem to involve specific brain networks and regions, as well as the activation of HPA axis, in the frame of abnormal response and activation to stress events [25]. Dysfunctional immune activation, as evidenced by plasma levels of immunoglobulins (Ig) or autoantibodies (autoAbs) reactive with neuropeptides and hormones, seems to relate with aggressive behaviors and psychiatric symptomatology [26]. Fetissov et al., for instance, found in individuals with eating disorders IgG reactive with melanocortin peptides alpha-melanocyte-stimulating hormone (α-MSH) and ACTH. Moreover, ACTH-reactive autoAbs have been observed in people with antisocial behavior [27]. At present, the effective role of autoAbs is still not clear, but these molecules react with peptides and hormones and may protect them from catabolism enhancing their biological function [28]. IgG autoAbs reacting with ACTH may be associated with significant aggressive conducts and antisocial behavior, further confirming this correlation.

A strong interaction takes place between the hypothalamus, the pituitary gland, and the adrenal cortex, leading to the secretion of different hormones. This axis represents the central coordinator of neuroendocrine reactions to stress and consists of the hypothalamic endocrinal component, the anterior portion of the pituitary gland, and an effector organ such the adrenal glands. Human behaviors, especially concerning aggressive conducts and danger perception, are strongly influenced by this neuroendocrine system whose effectors are hormones and peptides interacting at different levels and coordinating physiological reactions. Neuropeptides regulate physiological stress reaction involved in traumatic, allergic, and inflammatory events, developing long-term action contrary to neurotransmitters which operate in rapid times. Following a stressful event, paraventricular hypothalamic nuclei (PVN) secrete corticotropin-releasing hormone (CRH) which incomes directly in the hypothalamic-pituitary portal circulation. Paraventricular nuclei of the hypothalamus secrete CRH with 24 h daily variations, with highest levels in the morning and lower at night [29]. Adrenocorticotrophic hormone is subsequently secreted from anterior pituitary gland and stimulates glucocorticoids release from the adrenal glands. Glucocorticoids modulate metabolism, the immune system, and the central nervous system coordinating the physiological adaptive response to stress [30]. The main stimulus for ACTH synthesis and secretion comes from CRH, synergistically with arginine vasopressin (AVP) modulating effect; these modulators induce the release of ACTH from the storage systems in corticotropic neurons. ACTH induces the activation of intracellular signaling systems modulating adrenal cortisol synthesis in the adrenal cortex, in particular in its fasciculate and reticular zones. At present of our knowledge, a significant correlation between aggressiveness and violent behaviors on one side and ACTH secretion on the other one has been observed, with further confirmation from studies on ACTH autoAbs [31]. Interestingly, ACTH increases fighting conducts in mice, regardless to corticosterone release [32].

Different neural systems regulate the abovementioned axis, such as the prefrontal cortex and hippocampus which show an inhibiting action over the corticotrophin neurons of the hypothalamus, while the amygdala and the brainstem seem to activate these neurons. Glucocorticoids have a negative feedback over CRH neurons of PVN inhibiting its release. Glucocorticoids hypersecretion shows negative effects in respect to the hippocampus, leading to a reduction of dendritic spines and a neurogenesis impairment.

Cortisol represents the final step of the abovementioned axis: it is a steroid secreted from adrenal cortex during stress-related conditions influencing globally hormonal balance since cortisol receptors are present in several cells. Moreover, cortisol acts on blood sugar levels, physiological metabolism, anti-inflammatory effects, and creation of memory, in addition to its psychological implication as on anxiety and depression. Melanocyte-stimulating hormone (MSH) is another peptide hormone and neuropeptide synthetized in the brain by the pituitary gland consisting of different melanocortin peptides as α-MSH, β-MSH, and γ-MSH. It has been observed in experiments with mice that α-MSH is involved in stress-related externalizing behaviors and aggression, together with melanocortin peptides and ACTH fractions (amino acids 4–10) which, once released, induce aggressive conducts in mice [33]. It seems that the observed pro-aggressive ACTH effects require the melanocortin peptide pharmacophore. There is only two amino acids difference between the oxytocin (OT) and AVP sequences, which both consist of nine amino acid peptide hormones. OT has been observed having an influence at different levels; indeed, it modulates social and sexual behaviors and influences stress response [34, 35]. Moreover, it shows protective effects with regard to stress reactions; it modulates neural circuitry underlying social cognition processes and fear [36] and has been observed impairing the connection between the amygdala and brainstem effector nuclei of the autonomic nervous system in rats [37]. Interestingly, there is evidence of an intracerebral OT modulation inhibiting the activity of the HPA axis with neural and behavioral effects such as anxiety levels decrease [38, 39]. Therefore, it has been suggested that OT administration together with continuous social support may lead to anxiety levels reduction by the decrease of cortisol secretion [40]. Vasopressin (AVP) shows several functions among which aggressiveness neuromodulation that appear modulated in particular by the region of the central nervous system where this hormone is released. AVP is observed being stored with CRH in the same neurons [41], and together they induce ACTH-releasing activity [42]. Concerning the HPA axis, CRH represents the major stimulator for ACTH release during acute stress conditions. On the other hand, AVP shows an effect significantly considerable in chronic conditions [43].

Starting from the abovementioned considerations, a neurobiological model for stress-related brain's response, and subsequently derived behaviors and emotional reactions, such as anxiety, can be provided. Stress has been related to psychopathology, especially with regard to early rearing environment when it influences hormonal systems leading to later development of symptoms and determining specific behavioral patterns.

5.4 Techniques and Methods

The majority of critical situations may be contained and faced by a systematic interpersonal verbal approach, structured as a technique which can be applied in several different contexts and by different kinds of roles. For this reason, it appears fundamental to analyze the context in which de-escalation is required in order to clearly define the steps by which it may be possible to solve critical events.

Moreover, it appears useful to investigate some key concepts which co-occur in structuring potentially violent situations. Indeed, aggressive behaviors are characterized by an increased *arousal* which consists in psychomotor activation involving emotional, physical, and psychological changes. Furthermore, there is a systemic biological activation, involving the cardiovascular system, as well as the central, peripheral, and autonomic nervous system. These processes lead to an impairment of communication abilities and problem-solving capacities, which further exacerbate critical situations. Analyzing *aggressiveness escalation*, it appears clear that different steps contribute to violent behaviors. Indeed, different trigger factors could determinate psychophysical reactions leading to activated emotional conditions. A danger, both real and perceived, may appear as an imminent threat determining a maladaptive reaction characterized by the autonomic nervous system activation in presence of negative emotionality (fear and anger), psychomotor agitation, acute anxiety and distress, lowering of insight regarding action consequences, impulsivity, and hostile affect. Starting from this condition, *escalation* may lead to a point of no return in which violence is unavoidable, leading to actual crisis. Subsequently, a post-crisis phase has been described in which there is a resource exhaustion with mood deflection, establishing a condition of vulnerability to further violent episodes.

The abovementioned cycle could be interrupted only in the escalation phase which represent the last step in which a dialogical alliance may be possible. *De-escalation* is the technique of facing and interrupting emotional activation increase and potentially violent situations.

In this framework, de-escalation could be considered as a complex system of procedures and techniques aimed to desensitize individuals in order to contain and face the aggressiveness cycle in a particular relational context. It has been described as consisting of different aspects involving both verbal and nonverbal communication. De-escalation consists of functional and practical procedures which aim to establish a relationship with an agitated person, providing him the opportunity to calm down and resettle a functional emotional management. Therefore, when a person is pervaded by emotions such as anxiety and stress, he will reach a hyperactivated state of mind characterized by high internal energy (arousal), anxiety, disorientation, impaired reality judgment, behavioral problems, and impulse dyscontrol resulting in an overstimulated state of mind which represents a fragile condition prone to develop further emotional outbursts, leading to aggressive disruptions.

De-escalation is a relational methodology at the basis of functional dialogue and consists in the capacity of eliminating differences and disparities between people in different contexts. In order to build an effective and successful dialogue, reaching a mutual trust between parties, it is essential to deeply understand different roles and positions entering into a relationship. Furthermore, it appears fundamental to figure out the person we are talking with, his wishes, his desires, his worries and anxieties, and finally the problem he is facing.

De-escalation is conceived as the third step of the END method. To de-escalate means to reduce the level or intensity and to (cause to) become less dangerous or difficult in respect to an action or phenomenon which had intensified in a previous moment. In psychiatry and other medical contexts, the term de-escalation refers to a multitude of interventions based on elaborate verbal and nonverbal communication skills, techniques, and behavioral strategies employed by medical personnel in diverse situations in order to reduce the intensity of tension, anger, psychomotor agitation, and aggressiveness, or as preventative measure of aggressive or violent behavior. De-escalation is a means of desensitization with the objective of containing the natural course of the aggression cycle, and it should precede other potentially traumatizing measures such as rapid tranquillization, physical restraint, or seclusion, and only after its failure should these secondary interventions be applied.

The main purposes of the de-escalation process include a decrease in tension, fear, and aggressiveness, lowering the need for defensive attitude and the tendency to attack and eliminating triggers of aggressive and violent behavior while evaluating personal safety for oneself and those involved. De-escalation should create a suitable framework for dialogue and resolution, leaving a glimmer of possibility for initial collaboration, and eliminate confrontational and antagonistic positions similar to those of a win-lose situation. The de-escalation process, if adequate and effective, should last for a maximum of 10 min. To achieve the aforementioned results, multiple components (such as choice of words, personal mental state, posture, context) and particular procedures must be learned through specific training. There is not a strong evidence base supporting the de-escalation effectiveness due to the lack of randomized clinical trials which are complicated to conduct in the emergency settings where de-escalation is usually performed. For this reason, benefits for patients are relatively difficult to establish although it is rather clear and well documented that avoiding physical intervention is profitable both for medical staff and patients.

Effective communication techniques for de-escalation
- Avoid being rigid and antagonistic.
- Avoid contrapositions.
- Minimize any type of conflict.
- Search for a hint of collaboration and a starting point of understanding.
- Search for a point of agreement.
- Remain open to various possibilities.

Enhancing resilience before proceeding with de-escalation
- Assess your "power map": what can I do, what can the patient do, and what can others do.
- Proceed with context evaluation: potentially harmful objects, escape routes, and number of staff present.
- Assess help availability: assessment of the staff's competence to provide help if needed.
- Optimize your clinical knowledge of the patient: acquire preliminary information from medical personnel, family members, and clinical documentation before intervening (who is the patient, what did he "do" and why is he here, what have his reactions been like since his arrival).
- Evaluate personal emotional state: emotional reactivity, previous work load, fatigue, and type of interventions already performed.

When confronted with an agitated or potentially aggressive and violent patient
- Establish a relationship by introducing yourself and ask what (how?) would the other person prefer to be called.
- Ask concrete, open-ended questions and explain the reason why you are asking.
- Use short, clear sentences even at the expense of completeness.
- Find an agreement point.
- Teat the patient respectfully and cordially paying attention to the components of nonverbal communication such as voice tone, voice volume, and rhythm (prosody).
- Do not make assumptions about the patient's personality or life story.
- Use "I" statements which express your own thoughts rather than characteristics you attribute to the patient.
- Do not overpraise the patient; if appropriate pay a compliment inherent the conversation.
- Do not openly contradict the patient.
- Suggest alternatives and provide options.

Other more practical advice
- Speak softly with a calm tone of voice without yelling or raising your voice.
- Use appropriate language and vocabulary with respect to the person's sociocultural level.
- Do not talk over the patient.
- Ensure that you have been understood and that you have understood.
- Do not accuse, judge, or patronize.
- Do not respond in an aggressive manner.
- Offer something to eat or drink.
- Be respectful.
- Avoid phrases such as "no," "it's your fault," and "do you really need to do this?".
- Be comprehensive by using phrases such as "I understand, I'm sorry."
- Do not smile as it could be misinterpreted: the person could feel mocked.
- Avoid gesture which could seem arrogant or cocky (e.g., point a finger).
- Maintain eye contact occasionally shifting your glance.
- Maintain safety distance.
- Establish and maintain emotional contact and demonstrate emotional resonance.
- Avoid physical contact at any time.

Useful de-escalating phrases
- "It must be hard for you."
- "It happens to a lot of people we visit."
- "How did you get here? What can we do to help you?"
- "I am here, I am listening to you, I will try to help you within my possibilities."
- "What can I do for you?"
- "What worries you the most?"
- "Is there someone you trust that we could call?"
- "I agree with you up to a point."
- "I appreciate the fact that you accepted to talk with me."
- "We could decide to … for today."

Safety comes first
- In case of risk of violence, maintain at least a twice the arm's length physical distance.
- Position yourself so as to have an escape route behind your back.
- Do not constrain the patient with his back against the wall, or without any escape path.
- If there is any kind of weaponry, get away explaining that you do not feel comfortable and you do not accept to talk under these conditions.
- Avoid crossing your arms and keep them by your side with your palms open and facing forward.
- Make slow and steady gestures.

5.4.1 Risk Assessment

It appears fundamental to define specific factors that can provide reliable guidelines in order to prevent violent behaviors and aggressions as effectively as possible. Although there are no cues that can deterministically prevent future actions, specific signs may suggest the consequent urge of psychomotor agitation and violent conducts in relation to the current setting. More specifically, during patient's assessment, the ability to identify both objective and subjective signs which are suggestive of psychomotor agitation can significantly help in preventing escalation and aggressive manifestations. Being aware of such methodology not only appears fundamental to improve ability in de-escalation techniques and critical situations management of mental health operators, but it would also protect patient's health and integrity by preventing more dangerous situations and unpredictable complications.

The following are some points which should be kept in mind when assessing a patient in clinical settings and deciding how to approach him.

- Evaluate as thoroughly as possible the patient's history. Violence and aggressiveness are rarely unexpected since they are learned behaviors that provide violent people with feelings of power and self-confidence. Previous violent episodes may suggest the risk of further aggressive behaviors.
- Investigate bullying and history of violence which may lead to active repetition of such experiences. Furthermore, any domestic violence episodes or physical abuse has to be investigated since they may involve significant psychological consequences, in addition to a sort of "familiarity" to violence.
- Previous arrest or criminal conducts may suggest patient proneness to violence and antisocial behaviors.
- Investigate neurological problems and impulsive-compulsive disorders which may entail significant behavioral disorders concerning aggressiveness. These subjects are sensitive to frustration and show deficits in impulse control.
- Recent stressful events or significant losses may be risk factors for aggressiveness and violence.
- Drug and alcohol abuse is related to proneness to violence since it avoids inhibition systems leading to impulse control issues. Always investigate history of abuse and the possibility of an intoxication.
- Paranoid people, experiencing threat and persecutory ideation, may show low thresholds for acting violence.
- Severe psychopathological experiences may involve an increased risk of violence given the feeling of anguish they entail: command hallucinations may push people to act violently as well as mania in bipolar disorder can often manifest through aggressive behaviors.

The assessment phase has to be as forthcoming as possible, avoiding any stereotypical approach. At the same time, the interviewer should behave in a calm manner, subtly rejecting any possible manipulation by the interviewed. Direct questions do

Table 5.1 This table displays the most significant signals regarding risk assessment

Behavior	Language	Thought and perception	Space and borders	Context	Clinical status
Agitation, restlessness Rigid body posture Physical tension Threatening position Threatening stare	Verbal threats Insults Humiliations	Inability to concentration and focusing Disorganized thought Delusions of persecution and paranoia Hallucinations Disorientation and confusion	Patient feels invaded with regard to his space Patient invades other's space Patient claims that his requests are immediately met	Alcohol and drug abuse Previous violence signs Poor tolerance of frustration	Worsening of patient's mental state Poor insight and lack of collaboration Ineffectiveness of de-escalation strategies

not necessarily implicate an impersonal or judgmental approach. It is important to always bear in mind that the aim is to better understand how to help the interviewed patient. See the illustrative overview below (Table 5.1).

5.5 Clinical Examples

Behavioral manifestations are not always clearly distinguished from specific mental states. Indeed, an overlap between behavioral dysfunctions and different mental disorders is often observed. For example, a motor function independent from psychological dynamics determines behaviors and conducts. Moreover, a general approach is often required with regard to behavioral manifestations differing in their etiology, physiopathology, and neurobiological mechanism. Assuming this perspective, these behavioral features are considered as a whole leaving out distinctions about specific settings and treatments. As further support for such an approach, it is well-known that aggressiveness does not represent just a medical condition for which pharmacological interventions are the most suitable ones, but it also includes a well-defined psychological character which is fundamental to consider in order to intervene effectively. On the other side, agitation has too often been related to anxious states, not taking into account the possibility of non-linear correlations between externalized behavior and emotional distress: it is clear that agitated conducts not necessarily derive from psychological distress in a deterministic way. Starting from the abovementioned considerations, it appears fundamental to state that there is no psychiatric condition from which an episode of psychomotor agitation could not arise, at a different point of its course, from different trigger factors.

A well-defined approach to different clinical features appears fundamental in order to implement a suitable de-escalating procedure in our clinical practice.

Interestingly, about 6% of emergency room's accesses in the USA concern behavioral emergencies arising from mental health-related conditions [44]. In this frame, it appears that agitation and aggressiveness are the most relevant clinical aspects, both in psychiatric wards and in emergency settings. As stated before, the most common symptomatology consists of restlessness, psychomotor agitation, reactive mood and dysphoria, hyperarousal, and hyperexcitability [45]. Aggressiveness, both verbal and physical, may develop from these clinical conditions and is not always predictable. During an episode of psychomotor agitation, emotional contents could be overwhelming, becoming pervasive and dimming, without any possibility to control them and to manage frustration. Impressions and sensory stimuli can achieve a maddening level, and reciprocal communication can appear incomprehensible and interactions hostile, resulting in explicit outbursts and externalized behaviors. Violent behaviors have been found in 18.5% of recruited subjects in a systematic review about psychotic patients [1], stating that these dysfunctional conducts involve significant consequences for patients, caregivers, and healthcare operators who experience these stressful events leading to feelings of helplessness and frustration in addition to physical harm. Furthermore, this phenomenon leads to a worsening in stigmatization toward psychiatric illness and patients suffering from mental health problems. Up to date, in order to deal with episodes of psychomotor agitation and aggressive conducts, it is internationally recommended to employ de-escalation techniques and empathic communication procedures. Importantly, feasibility and opportunity for this kind of intervention have to be accurately evaluated by clinicians or operators who have to manage these situations. It is not always possible to proceed with communicative methods given the total inability to build a cooperative dialogue with individuals agitated and emotionally overwhelmed. For these reasons, in the event that communication is deemed not viable or ineffective, the need for pharmacological tranquillization significantly emerges, as stated by the most reliable international guidelines (NICE 2019). When pharmacological approach is not feasible, seclusion (involuntary placement of a patient in a bounded area that he cannot leave) or restraints (involuntary mechanical and physical restriction in order to manage an agitated patient) could be used in several clinical settings. In this regard, pharmacological protocols and intervention procedures from randomized controlled trials have been systematically reviewed in order to set up shared and reliable guidelines, but this argument exceeds these chapter's targets.

In regard to what a clinician may be required to deal with in his working setting, it is fundamental to underline that any kind of approach cannot neglect the need of a state diagnosis in order to effectively intervene. Therefore, communication techniques are addressed to behavioral manifestations, symptomatic features, and dimensional description, at first overshadowing the inner psychopathological experience of the patient. In the context of emergency settings, what clinicians are required to face are urgent situations needing effective approach in order to avoid aggressive behaviors with actual physical violence toward oneself, others, property, or verbal threats. From this perspective, any kind of agitated conduct and even more so specific aggressive and violent episodes has to be considered, first and foremost, as a medical emergency until causes such as delirium, metabolic, or infectious disorders have been ruled out. Agitated individuals can behave violently for different reasons, and they can suffer from different disorders, all potentially leading to dysfunctional manifestations. What we would like to underline here is that in any case we are arguing about a question of dysfunctional communication, involving the urge from these subjects of venting frustration, fear, and distress. In some way, these individuals are willing to be heard, and, even if in a dysfunctional way and sometimes violently, they are seeking to communicate and are looking for someone able to understand and take care of them. Bearing these considerations in mind, our goal is to dig deeper and analyze more closely specific clinical settings which health workers are very often supposed to face. What we would like to propose is a dimensional approach to empathic communication and de-escalation techniques. As said before, in clinical settings the main aim is to face as soon as possible behaviors and conducts arising from emotional dimensions and abnormal feelings. Given the fact that the above-mentioned overwhelming emotional states seem to be shared among nosography and categorical diagnosis, only a dimensional approach would be truly effective. In this way it is possible to manage behaviors regardless of psychopathology and course which would require more time and deeper analysis in order to be reliable.

5.5.1   The Disorganized Patient

There are several conditions leading to disorganization which is represented by the inability for the subject to adequately set up and organize ideas, thoughts, and emotional contents. The patient seems unable to focus on the surrounding reality, without any capacity to distinguish the foreground from the background of the present context; it is not possible to build a logical reasoning which could be shared, starting from common sense. The ability to relate with others is impaired, given the presence of illogical and unintelligible thought. Disorganized patients can be overwhelmed by "normal" communication which could appear incomprehensive and hostile. Furthermore, they can be unable to manage frustration and feelings, as well as being scared by perceptions and sensory impressions which can appear abnormally vivid and overwhelming. People with cognitive deficits may present an impairment of their problem-solving abilities, showing significant deficits in managing emotional frustration, experiencing profound anxiety, and potentially manifesting outbursts.
    To effectively communicate with these subjects, it is recommended to:

- Simplify as much as possible the communication dividing sentences in very small and elementary parts. Small tasks and easy instructions can be more understandable by helping to focus attention.
- Repeat several times your statement, using the same words. Employing more expressive words appears useless. Repetition may appear as a reference point, helping to orientate and focus cognition.
- Avoid any kind of intimidation, anger, or subjective frustration which will worsen attempts, making things harder. Emotional modulation of nonverbal communication is not recommended since disorganized people will be inclined to misunderstand it.
- Employ positive reinforcements which may be perceived as significant motivating feedback.

5.5.2 The Psychotic Patient

From a descriptive point of view, psychotic patients present delusions and halluci-nations, often in addition to disorganized thoughts and behaviors. This clinical symptomatology makes communicative attempts very hard given the fact that these patients are uncompromising and adamant about their beliefs. Delusional patients are willing to convince others about their absolute convictions, and any attempt aimed to set up a "logical reasoning" with them will inevitably fail. More specifi-cally, psychotic patients may appear autistic, given the tendency to live in their own world being auto-referential and unable to establish a relationship based on com-mon sense. In particular, their ability to steer relations and conversations toward stability zones, which are shared logical points allowing to "get in touch" with the interlocutor, appears significantly impaired.

To effectively communicate with these subjects, it is recommended to:

- Avoid long and complex discussion which may only reinforce delusional beliefs. In front of strongly built and cemented delusions, the main aim is to disengage. It is absolutely not recommended to attempt to convince a delusional subject that his beliefs are not true. The risk is to elicit anger and frustration worsening even more such a tough situation.
- Try to steer discussion toward arguments in regard to which the patient does not seem delusional. Whenever possible, this kind of approach may calm down the setting, engaging the patient and allowing a more peaceful exchange with him.
- Investigate with a mild approach the delusional content, in order to evaluate its pervasiveness and its potential consequences about self-harm or intention to hurt other people. Avoid agreeing with delusions and hallucinations since it will only strengthen their structure.
- Whenever possible, try to argue about delusions and hallucinations' reality with the patient as to provide a reality support which may help him.
- In most cases, it could be helpful to distinguish the patient's point of view and experience from yours: carefully describe yourself as skeptical and state that you think he is truly perceiving what he is describing and that his own convictions could be real even if you do not believe it, at least for now. One can remain strictly convinced of his own beliefs even if they are not shared.
- Pay attention to what the patient is saying and show that you are doing so. Kindly interrupt the patient when his speech is disorganized and tangential. Try to sum up his arguments and reorganize them, providing the impression that you are actively participating in the discussion.
- Try to keep the environment familiar and safe, avoiding any trouble or interrup-tion which may worse the patient's agitation. Do not stand too close to the patient, limit eye contact, and avoid as much as possible physical contact.

5.5.2.1 Clinical Example

Gino is a 47 years old man who was born and grew up in Rome. He dropped out of school due to his illness. In the past, he worked on some occasions as a mechanic always having difficulties with his duties. Gino believes he is a "space agent of Carabinieri Headquarters (Italian Police Force)" with the identification code 180–180–180 (180×3). He has a special mission he is not allowed to talk about. He says he needs to go to Dusseldorf in Germany where an intergalactic Starfleet Carabinieri will take off. He absolutely needs to talk to the Supreme Pontiff in order to get official permission to participate in the mission. Gino was accompanied to the emergency room by his brother because he was getting progressively agitated and anxious at home. The on-call psychiatrist was called to manage the situation.

- Gino: "Doctor, you cannot understand, that's normal, but I have to go, the Pope is waiting for me. It will be a mess if I don't!"
- Doctor: "You are right, I don't get the point actually. Would you like to explain to me what's going on?"
- G: "Come on, don't be so boring, just let me go!"
- D: "Gino, I do not want to bother you, I do not understand, and I would like to … why is the Pope waiting for you? Are you sure? I guess that he will be very busy, he is the Pope! Let's get in that room, just to talk a bit. Maybe we'll find out how to solve this problem together."
- G:"You cannot."
- D: "Maybe, but I would like to try … is there something that is scaring you? Or something that you cannot talk about? You are not obliged to tell me everything. We can just try to find a solution, don't you think?"
- G: "Please, give up. It's about something enormous, something huge. About an intergalactic mission that I am supposed to participate to … but I cannot say more, please."
- D: "That's great! It seems really interesting! You know, I was a huge fan of Buzz Lightyear when I was young, "to infinity and beyond!""
- G: "Oh, come on, you don't believe me?"
- D: "Gino, I am just trying to understand what you are saying and I would like to hear more from you, really."
- G: "But do you think I am lying?"
- D: "I do believe that you are talking about something extremely important for you and that's the reason why I would like to further discuss it with you. I would really like to help you. But I think that at the moment it won't be possible for you to go to the Vatican"
- G: "Why?"
- D: "Because it is late, and you seem a bit worried. The Pope won't welcome you now, that's pretty sure. He goes to bed very early. I think it would be better for you to take some time off in the forthcoming days. You need some rest and we may try to talk a bit about all that stuff … do you agree?"
- G: "I need a shower."
- D: "That's true …"
- G: "I cannot show up in front of the Pope in these conditions."
- D: "We'll think about all of that. So, are you in?"

- G: "Yeah ok. But just for a few days. In 2 weeks' time it will be Easter and the Pope will be busy, I am sure."
- D: "You're right. Ok let's go."
- G: "Let me tell you something, I don't want your disgusting soup ok? I hate it! I won't eat it, ok?"
- D: "Ok Gino, don't worry … only pasta for you …"

5.5.3 The Manic Patient

A manic patient shows high energy level, psychomotor agitation, and excited and/or irritable mood, requires little sleep, and has accelerated and chaotic ideation with disorganized thoughts and a cascade of words. He is energetic, abnormally self-confident, and grandiose, showing a sense of invulnerability which often leads to dangerous actions and behaviors. In most severe cases, the patient becomes psychotic and delusional, manifesting megalomaniac and persecutory ideation, and often uses drugs, both to sustain his excited state and to calm down.

To effectively communicate with these subjects, it is recommended to:

- Remain calm and concentrated. Avoid any involvement with regard to the manipulative approach of the patients who can be provocative and attractive, resorting in some cases to sexualized interactions.
- Speak slowly and use simple and easily understandable statements, trying to slow down the interaction. Agitation feeds itself with agitation.
- Be empathic and comprehensive, taking into account that behind the grandiosity and the self-confidence there is a profound sense of vulnerability as the psychological core of this condition. Therefore, avoid direct and blunt communication.
- Underline whenever possible the importance of a regular compliance to pharmacotherapy in order to establish an ordinary everyday lifestyle.

5.5.3.1 Clinical Example

Franco is a 50-year-old Italian man. He is divorced and has two children. He loves cycling and playing bridge. He has a bachelor's degree in economics. He has no history of drug or alcohol abuse he has changed jobs many times, and on some occasions got fired, due to his mental disorder: Franco has suffered from bipolar disorder type I since the age of 28. When going into manic episode, he feels rested after only 2 h of sleep at night, he becomes extremely euphoric and talkative, his thoughts are racing leading eventually to tangentiality and derailment, and he can cycle for hours covering huge distances without stopping to rest. He gradually starts manifesting grandiose delusions stating he is God. Franco was accompanied to the emergency room by his ex-wife because he was getting extremely euphoric and delusional; he had gambled thousands of euros playing bridge the week before; he hadn't been sleeping for 3 days, and on that same day, he had also cycled for 8 h without showing any signs of fatigue. The on-call psychiatrist was called to manage this episode of full-blown mania.

- Franco: "Good evening Doctor, how are you? You seem a little tired, I don't understand why they had to call you at 03:00 a.m. I actually don't understand why I'm even here in the first place. I feel perfectly fine, full of energy and so happy. Since I wanted to get out of the house I agreed to accompany my ex-wife. I actually thought we were gonna get some ice cream. I love ice cream, especially fruit flavours. Fruit is actually very good for your health, during summer it helps you hydrate even more. Oooh summer finally, I can't wait to go on vacation, I will do as I like and nobody will bother me. Where did you go on vacation last summer?"
- Doctor: "Mr. Franco, my name is Mario Rossi, I am a psychiatrist. I was called because my colleague and your ex-wife, who has known you for 30 years, think that you are not well."
- F: "That's ridiculous, I've never felt better. I cycled for 8 h straight today. Did you know I won the world cycling championship this year? What time is it? I should start my morning exercise in a while."
- D: "Mr. Franco, as a psychiatrist I must tell you that it seems you are not well. Sometimes feeling this great can be pathological. I was told you suffer from Bipolar Disorder and that you are under treatment, is that right?"
- F: "Yes, but this is different. What you are saying is nonsense. It has nothing to do with this bipolar disease. I stopped taking this lithium rubbish and I've never felt better, maybe I'm not even bipolar and doctors like you had it wrong all this time."
- D: "Mr. Franco, I understand that right now what I'm saying seems nonsense right now but"
- F: "There is no but, it's just nonsense."
- D: "Mr. Franco, please just hear me out, my only interest is helping you. No sleeping without signs of fatigue, extreme gambling, constant euphoria end excitement, you have had episodes like this in the past."
- F: "Yes I have, but this is no episode."
- D: "We cannot be sure of that. If it is an episode a tremendous depression could follow, as I was told has happened in the past, and it would be the price to pay for not having accepted psychiatric help right now."
- F: "Psychiatric help means being injected drugs forcefully and being tied up in bed and staying hospitalized for a month for no reason."
- D: "I'm very sorry that you had to undergo such a traumatizing experience but I assume that things were out of control and my colleagues had to intervene mandatorily to preserve your own and others' safety."
- F: "I was feeling super even at that time."
- D: "Mr. Franco, I think that the best solution would be a voluntary stay in our psychiatric ward so as to avoid both a mandatory stay in the near future or a subsequent depressive episode."
- F: "A month away? I have a thousand things to do!!"
- D: "If you accept to stay now your hospitalization will definitely last less than a month. We have to find the right stabilizing cure and help you get lots of sleep."

- F: "Maybe 3 days without sleeping is a bit much although I feel great. I understand that at some point I will have to sleep ..."
- D: "So do you agree?"
- F: "Yes, are you sure that things are going to go the way you promised?"
- D: "You have my word!"
- F: "Can I have coffee during the stay?"
- D: "Only decaffeinated coffee, those are the rules for all the patients."
- F: "I guess I can live with that ..."

5.5.4 The Angry Patient

In front of an angry person, it is fundamental to avoid further escalation leading to an enraged state which is likely to provoke violence and aggressive conducts. Therefore, it is necessary to achieve emotional stability before approaching and trying to control the setting and the environment. There is no way to face reasons and causes of anger without an effective control strategy aimed to avoid a worsening of such a critical situation. Always try to rule out intoxication or medical conditions which could underlie these behaviors. Angry people are suffering, moved by a profound anguish, overwhelmed by their feelings, and stressed by their inability to correctly communicate them. These considerations, once again, appear fundamental in approaching techniques.

To effectively communicate with these subjects, it is recommended to:

- Assure safety for yourself and others in order to be able to assist and effectively intervene.
- Disengage from the competitive approach of angry people. They will refuse any kind of negotiation and compromise, trying to overwhelm you in order to get what they want. It is not worth arguing about the content of their request before calming down their agitated mental state. Be empathic but not compassionate; whenever possible provide positive reinforcements and slow down the interaction.
- Be careful and attentive, showing your interest in what the interlocutor is saying and about his concerns. Pay attention and try to focus on what is generating anxiety, even without initially deepening patient's concerns in an explicit way: just your presence and the fact that you are paying attention can be helpful; angry people often calm down autonomously.
- Behave the same way you want others to behave. Speak calmly, briefly, and with simple statements. Do not act impulsively and do not assume threatening postures. In these cases, people may be conditioned to imitate your behavior.

Red-hot rage implies a reactive and coordinated behavior aimed to hurt and hit others; it entails a higher arousal and an excited mind state which makes very tough to interact with people in such condition. In this state, individuals do not think about consequences of their actions, since they are looking for an immediate reward. They do not feel guilty, and they feel comfortable in this excited condition. These individuals desire rage and excitement, and they look for intensity and action, experiencing them as the normal effect of frustration. When facing such a person, who is no longer trying to communicate with you but only threatening and being aggressive, it could be helpful to briefly communicate essential and imperative statements, consisting of few simple words, with regard to their current dangerous behavior, asking to the person to immediately "cease and desist." Repeat your statement until this behavior is interrupted. In this case, do not use scolding tones and try to appear uncompromising. In order to effectively de-escalate an interaction with an enraged person, it is important to avoid any public statement pointing out the person's fears and weakness areas. In this way people will appear less reluctant to dialogue. Moreover, it could be helpful to leave them with the impression that they have the last word, since their need to appear as unafraid and feel listened will be respected. Finally, in front of predatory individuals, who display deliberate intimidation and aggressiveness, in a cold and psychopathic manner, it is essential to guarantee yours and other operators' safety. These individuals are willing to prevail over other people, and they are prepared to do anything in order to impose their own interests. It is important to appear self-confident and firm; appear insensitive to intimidations and harassments, since these individuals will probably not be interested in someone who does not appear as the "next victim." It is fundamental to avoid body movements, posture, or the tone of voice that may elicit aggressive behaviors, always being prepared to this eventuality. Remind that there will be the consequences to their actions, with clear and simple statements regarding the possible law implications of their behavior. The only aim of such a strategy is to demotivate these individuals so that they do not act violently. The most effective approach in this kind of situation is stating that you will not accept intimidation or aggressiveness, appearing as someone not worth to victimize. In these cases, negotiation will not be effective since they will consider it as a confirmation of weakness as well as a further incentive to prevail and overwhelm the interlocutor.

5.5.5 The Patient with Suicidal Ideation

For any mental health operator, suicidal ideation is one of the most complex situations he is required to deal with, being a frustrating and destabilizing event. It is really hard to imagine that suicide could be considered as a valid option for someone who is experiencing an endless and hopeless pain. Unfortunately, there are conditions in regard to which psychological sufferance becomes unbearable and no longer acceptable, rendering individuals unable to conceive an alternative or at least an end to their pain, besides suicide. In literature, several risk factors for suicide have been described: demographic data, gender, ethnicity, educational and economic status, family history for mental illness, and previous suicide attempts. Nevertheless, it becomes increasingly clear that suicide has an unpredictable character. Suicidal ideation arises from different psychopathological milieu. The approach to such a condition needs particular intervention strategies that appear valid regardless of the categorical diagnosis. Furthermore, it appears important to consider psychological processes underlying self-harm intentions besides proper suicidal ideation.

To effectively communicate with these subjects, it is recommended to:

- Try to approach the person in a calm environment where you are able to intervene without interruptions. However, it is important to avoid an isolated environment since violence is unpredictable.
- Pay attention to your behavior: eye contact should be occasional, representing a moment of confidentiality. Your approach has to be moderate, avoiding dramatic tones without rejecting the patient's suffering. Be empathic and comprehensive but not excessively confidential since it could seem inauthentic.
- In most cases, avoid direct communication: try to engage the patient by talking about "lighter" and less demanding arguments before exploring their emotional contents.
- Avoid an excessively hesitant approach. People with suicidal ideation can find maddening a passive intervention which may further distance the patient from the alliance with the operator. In front of a concrete suicidal project, do not hesitate to ask direct questions about the patient's intentions: this intervention can often relieve patients form their inner anguish given their difficulty to communicate such a content.
- Manage your own emotions and worries, without showing your nervousness. These patients are hopeless and overwhelmed, but they are highly sensitive, and they will not trust you if you do not appear sufficiently reliable with regard to such a situation. Use a calm and stable tone of voice and try to appear self-confident. These patients need to feel that you can handle the situation.
- Always bear in mind that you are not almighty: provide all your competence and your professionalism doing your best to rescue these people. Consider such conditions in the perspective of possibilities and not of failures.
- Remember that even if you are not providing direct solutions to the problem, simply talking about it can have a healing effect. Dialogue keeps people away from suicide, making them more available to de-escalation. Individuals will feel more worthy and deserving and less isolated and alone, given the presence of someone who cares about them.

5.5.5.1 Clinical Example

Laura is a 26-year-old law student, studying away from home. She is an only child, and her parents have high expectations of her. She recently broke up with her boyfriend of 3 years. She has no personal history of drug and alcohol abuse or mental disorder, but there is family history for mood disorders. Laura, already late in terms of graduation and still having to sustain six important exams, has found herself caught up in a spiral of lies: her parents think that she is going to graduate in a month. Laura was accompanied to the emergency room by her best friend after having asked for her help since she had been feeling depressed, anxious, and suicidal during the last week. The on-call psychiatrist was called to manage the situation.

- Doctor: "Good evening Laura. My name is Mario Rossi, I'm a psychiatrist and I was called to offer my help. How are you feeling? What can I do for you?"
- Laura: (crying) "Hi, I am feeling terrible, I am desperate and I can't take it anymore. I don't know if there is anything you can do to help me."
- D: "I'm really sorry that you feel this way. Would you like to explain what is going on so maybe we can find together a way that I can help you."
- L: "I'm a failure, my parents think I'm graduating from law school next month but it's not true. I want all this to end, just to end …"
- D: "Law school, wow, it must be very hard. Do you like it?"
- L: "I'm not sure, I thought I did but if I really did I would have already graduated …"
- D: "Laura, I can understand how that feels but it's not a race. It also took me 2 years more to graduate from medical school."
- L: "I should have studied more, I know I should have, I'm a failure …"
- D: "What did you mean before when you said that you want this to end? Have you ever thought of death as a possible solution?"
- L: (crying) "I have, I don't know what to do, my parents will be devastated if they learn about the truth."
- D: "Laura, they will be much more devastated if you are dead. Listen to me, as a psychiatrist I have never come across a single suicide attempt survivor who was not grateful for having survived."
- L: "But what do I do? Every choice seems like a dead end … at least if I'm dead I won't feel so dreadful anymore and I can finally rest …"
- D: "Laura, please listen to me, you're in a very bad place right now and everything seems impossible. You are severely depressed and unfortunately there is no room for positive and optimistic thoughts in your mind."
- L: "No, there isn't because there is no such possibility."
- D: "Let us take care of you. I'm just asking you to undergo a hospital stay in order to try and fix this situation together."
- L: "And how am I supposed to fix this?"
- D: "We need to talk about this whole situation, understand how you got here. Afterwards we can organize a visit for your parents where we will all talk together and you can finally reveal this "secret". You should also take medication for some time, we will talk about it in the ward. What do you think?"
- L: "I don't know what else to do, maybe I should try out what you're suggesting."
- D: "I think you should, you're not the first student that comes in the emergency room with such a problem and all others have gone on with their life after their hospital stay."
- L: "Ok …"

5.5.6 The Patient Suffering Severe Withdrawal from Intoxicating Substances

This clinical situation has to be considered a full-fledged medical emergency, and therefore it is always fundamental to bear in mind that de-escalation has a marginal role. In such cases, the main point is to alert emergency services or to treat intoxication. People in withdrawal are agitated and restless, making hard to get in touch with them. Moreover, a mental disorder is often simultaneously present in the context of a dual diagnosis, significantly complicating the handling of the situation: substance abuse worsens clinical features, and mental illness makes harder substances dependency management.

In order to manage a withdrawal syndrome, while waiting for medical assistance, keep in mind the following points:

- The patient could be disoriented and unstable and often confused, given the lowering of consciousness and vigilance. In that case, try putting him in a safe place in order to protect him.
- Their sensorial and receptive functions are impaired; therefore, try to avoid any overwhelming stimuli in order to avert impulsive and aggressive behavior. Speak clearly and simply. Avoid sudden movements since they could elicit a startle reflex or an unpredictable reaction.
- Patients in withdrawal could also be angry and violent and aggressive. De-escalate the interaction bearing in mind that they are suffering from a medical condition and are often not aware of the situation. Pay attention and listen in a comprehensive way, all the while reassuring them.

5.6 Conclusions

For any mental health operator, dealing with crisis situations and agitated people who are emotionally overwhelmed represents a possible occurrence. Therefore, it is important to be prepared in order to manage such situations in the best possible way. It is fundamental to know how to approach agitated people, being able to manage situations which can suddenly worsen. There are several clinical conditions which include aggressive behaviors. More precisely, any kind of mental issues may occasionally lead to dysfunctional conducts which seem to share the urge to communicate emotional contents, even though with the due differences. Becoming aware of the inability to communicate their emotionality gives rise to frustration and more proneness to aggressive behavior. Starting from these considerations, it appears clear that any operator who is supposed to deal with such clinical circumstances should develop communication techniques and de-escalation abilities aimed to effectively manage critical situations and prevent higher critical interactions or physical aggressions. De-escalation is conceived as the set of techniques aimed to desensitize agitation and interrupt the aggressiveness cycle. These techniques employ both verbal and nonverbal procedures [46]. In this frame, we sought to provide effective guidelines and rational protocols, based on communication techniques, which could assist anyone operating in emergency settings. However, it is clear that dealing with psychomotor agitation and unpredictable behaviors, self-control is involved. Mental health operators' ability to stay calm and manage circumstances from a psychological point of view becomes fundamental. We are not arguing about an enforced sense of control, but on the contrary, we described a fluid mental state allowing to adequately adapt our conditions to the context: starting from the capacity to accurately recognize a potentially dangerous situation by being aware of its potential development, we should be able to a purposeful and helpful approach. Self-confidence is about awareness of one's own limits as well as one's own experience and abilities. A de-escalation approach does not have to be influenced by other's anguish or hurry. Such an attitude requires time, displaying reassuring reliability, in order effectively manage crisis situations. It is important to assume a reassuring body language, managing fears and emotions, respecting distances, and displaying empathic communication. This attitude will be able to manage overt hostility and fear manifestations. These specific indications should be assumed in order to avoid a competitive dynamic where hostility grows further [13]. Indeed, during an intervention, it is important to bear in mind that the main aim is to build an equitable dialogue in order to listen and try to give answers. It would be totally inappropriate to turn a clinical interview into a competitive striving for "the truth," risking to elicit an endless dispute and losing sight of the main purpose. It is clear how any answer in kind would be counterproductive in dealing with insults and provocation, definitively compromising the relationship. In particular, any kind of disparaging attack should not be taken personally due to the fact that it belongs to a specific context: although such situations are without doubt difficult and demeaning, by being resilient and context-appropriate, one should be able to confront the situation. For anyone who is supposed to deal with such complex situations, it is important to develop self-knowledge, taking into account one's own vulnerabilities. Dealing with agitated and aggressive people, as described in the present chapter, represents a fundamental ability in clinical practice, especially in the context of emergency rooms which are not always adequately equipped to effectively manage psychiatric conditions and their acute manifestations, such as psychomotor agitation, due to different difficulties: understaffed or not properly trained personnel, uncontrolled rooms where patients may be left unattended and free to get blunt objects which could be used in self-harm or suicide attempts, lack of structured risk assessment functional to a correct dealing with agitated or intoxicated patients, and poor screening tools. Moreover, these patients remain too often unobserved in emergency room until they represent an actual issue, displaying aggressiveness or behaving violently. Therefore, it is fundamental to implement specific interventions aimed to reduce these obstacles regarding clinical practice. We are convinced of the importance of a cultural change in order to eliminate any kind of stigma with regard to individuals suffering from mental disorders who, despite their explicit behaviors, are actually fragile and deeply suffering.

References

1. Witt K, van Dorn R, Fazel S. Risk factors for violence in psychosis: systematic review and meta-regression analysis of 110 studies [published correction appears in PLoS One. 2013;8(9). doi:10.1371/annotation/f4abfc20-5a38-4dec-aa46-7d28018bbe38]. PLoS One. 2013;8(2):e55942. https://doi.org/10.1371/journal.pone.0055942.
2. Iozzino L, Ferrari C, Large M, Nielssen O, de Girolamo G. Prevalence and risk factors of violence by psychiatric acute inpatients: a systematic review and meta-analysis. PLoS One. 2015;10(6):e0128536. https://doi.org/10.1371/journal.pone.0128536.
3. Ziaei M, Massoudifar A, Rajabpour-Sanati A, Pourbagher-Shahri AM, Abdolrazaghnejad A. Management of violence and aggression in emergency environment; a narrative review of 200 related articles. Adv J Emerg Med. 2018;3(1):e7. https://doi.org/10.22114/AJEM. v0i0.117.
4. Clements PT, DeRanieri JT, Clark K, Manno MS, Kuhn DW. Workplace violence and corporate policy for health care settings. Nurs Econ. 2005;23(3):119–24, 07.
5. Gerberich SG, Church TR, McGovern PM, Hansen H, Nachreiner NM, Geisser MS, et al. Risk factors for work-related assaults on nurses. Epidemiology. 2005;16(5):704–9.
6. Van Dorn R, Volavka J, Johnson N. Mental disorder and violence: is there a relationship beyond substance use? Soc Psychiatry Psychiatr Epidemiol. 2012;47(3):487–503. https://doi. org/10.1007/s00127-011-0356-x.
7. Whittington R, Richter D. From the individual to the interpersonal: environment and interaction in the escalation of violence in mental health settings. In: Richter D, Whittington R, editors. Violence in mental health settings: causes, consequences, management. New York, NY: Springer Science + Business Media; 2006. p. 47–65. https://doi.org/10.1007/978-0-387-33965-8_3.
8. Elbogen EB, Johnson SC. The intricate link between violence and mental disorder: results from the national epidemiologic survey on alcohol and related conditions. Arch Gen Psychiatry. 2009;66(2):152–61. https://doi.org/10.1001/archgenpsychiatry.2008.537.
9. National Institute for Clinical Excellence (NICE). Violence and aggression: short-term management in mental health, health and community settings. London: NICE; 2015. https://www. nice.org.uk/guidance/ng10. Accessed June 2019.
10. Allen JJ, Anderson CA, Bushman BJ. The general aggression model. Curr Opin Psychol. 2018;19:75–80. https://doi.org/10.1016/j.copsyc.2017.03.034.
11. Lukens TW, Wolf SJ, Edlow JA, et al. Clinical policy: critical issues in the diagnosis and management of the adult psychiatric patient in the emergency department. Ann Emerg Med. 2006;47:79–99.
12. Andrade C. Rapid tranquillisation in emergency psychiatric settings. BMJ. 2007;335(7625):835–6. https://doi.org/10.1136/bmj.39359.614387.80.
13. Amdur E. Grace under fire: skills for calming and de-escalating aggressive and mentally ill individuals. 2nd ed. Shoreline, WA: Edgework Books; 2011.
14. Kaplan SG, Wheeler EG. Survival skills for working with potentially violent clients. Social Casework. 1983;64(6):339–46.
15. Nelson RJ, Trainor BC. Neural mechanisms of aggression. Nat Rev Neurosci. 2007;8(7):536–46. https://doi.org/10.1038/nrn2174.
16. Wrangham RW. Two types of aggression in human evolution. Proc Natl Acad Sci. 2018;115(2):245–53. https://doi.org/10.1073/pnas.1713611115.
17. Keynejad RC, Frodl T, Kanaan R, Pariante C, Reuber M, Nicholson TR. Stress and functional neurological disorders: mechanistic insights. J Neurol Neurosurg Psychiatry. 2019;90(7):813–21. https://doi.org/10.1136/jnnp-2018-318297.
18. Veenema AH, Torner L, Blume A, Beiderbeck DI, Neumann ID. Low inborn anxiety correlates with high intermale aggression: link to ACTH response and neuronal activation of the hypothalamic paraventricular nucleus. Horm Behav. 2007;51(1):11–9. https://doi.org/10.1016/j. yhbeh.2006.07.004.

19. Chrousos GP, Gold PW. The concepts of stress and stress system disorders. Overview of physical and behavioral homeostasis. JAMA. 1992;267(9):1244–52. https://doi.org/10.1001/jama.1992.03480090092034.

20. van Honk J, Peper JS, Schutter DJ. Testosterone reduces unconscious fear but not consciously experienced anxiety: implications for the disorders of fear and anxiety. Biol Psychiatry. 2005;58(3):218–25. https://doi.org/10.1016/j.biopsych.2005.04.003.

21. Haller J, Mikics E, Halasz J, Toth M. Mechanisms differentiating normal from abnormal aggression: glucocorticoids and serotonin. Eur J Pharmacol. 2005;526(1–3):89–100. https://doi.org/10.1016/j.ejphar.2005.09.064.

22. Reardon AF, Hein CL, Wolf EJ, Prince LB, Ryabchenko K, Miller MW. Intermittent explosive disorder: associations with PTSD and other Axis I disorders in a US military veteran sample. J Anxiety Disord. 2014;28(5):488–94. https://doi.org/10.1016/j.janxdis.2014.05.001.

23. Hökfelt T, Bartfai T, Bloom F. Neuropeptides: opportunities for drug discovery. Lancet Neurol. 2003;2(8):463–72. https://doi.org/10.1016/S1474-4422(03)00482-4.

24. Lin D, Boyle MP, Dollar P, Lee H, Lein E, Perona P, et al. Functional identification of an aggression locus in the mouse hypothalamus. Nature. 2011;470(7333):221. https://doi.org/10.1038/nature09736.

25. Summers CH, Winberg S. Interactions between the neural regulation of stress and aggression. J Exp Biol. 2006;209(23):4581–9. https://doi.org/10.1242/jeb.02565.

26. Vaeroy H, Schneider F, Fetissov SO. Neurobiology of aggressive behavior-role of autoantibodies reactive with stress-related peptide hormones. Front Psych. 2019;10:872. https://doi.org/10.3389/fpsyt.2019.00872.

27. Fetissov SO, Hallman J, Nilsson I, Lefvert AK, Oreland L, Hökfelt T. Aggressive behavior linked to corticotropin-reactive autoantibodies. Biol Psychiatry. 2006;60(8):799–802. https://doi.org/10.1016/j.biopsych.2006.03.081.

28. Takagi K, Legrand R, Asakawa A, Amitani H, François M, Tennoune N, et al. Anti-ghrelin immunoglobulins modulate ghrelin stability and its orexigenic effect in obese mice and humans. Nat Commun. 2013;4(2685):1–11. https://doi.org/10.1038/ncomms3685.

29. Dutt M, Jialal I. Physiology, adrenal gland. StatPearls. Bethesda, MD: StatPearls Publishing; 2019.

30. Allen MJ, Sharma S. StatPearls. In: Physiology, adrenocorticotropic hormone (ACTH). Bethesda, MD: StatPearls Publishing; 2019.

31. Vaeroy H, Adori C, Legrand R, Lucas N, Breton J, Cottard C, et al. Autoantibodies reactive to adrenocorticotropic hormone can alter cortisol secretion in both aggressive and nonaggressive humans. Proc Natl Acad Sci U S A. 2018;115(28):E6576–e6584. https://doi.org/10.1073/pnas.1720008115.

32. Brain PF, Evans AE. Acute influences of some ACTH-related peptides of fighting and adrenocortical activity in male laboratory mice. Pharmacol Biochem Behav. 1977;7(5):425–33. https://doi.org/10.1016/0091-3057(77)90210-6.

33. Nowell N, Thody A, Woodley R. α-Melanocyte stimulating hormone and aggressive behavior in the male mouse. Physiol Behav. 1980;24(1):5–9. https://doi.org/10.1016/0031-9384(80)90006-2.

34. Campbell A. Oxytocin and human social behavior. Pers Soc Psychol Rev. 2010;14(3):281–95. https://doi.org/10.1177/1088868310363594.

35. Stoop R. Neuromodulation by oxytocin and vasopressin. Neuron. 2012;76(1):142–59. https://doi.org/10.1016/j.neuron.2012.09.025.

36. Kirsch P, Esslinger C, Chen Q, Mier D, Lis S, Siddhanti S, et al. Oxytocin modulates neural circuitry for social cognition and fear in humans. J Neurosci. 2005;25(49):11489–93. https://doi.org/10.1523/JNEUROSCI.3984-05.2005.

37. Huber D, Veinante P, Stoop R. Vasopressin and oxytocin excite distinct neuronal populations in the central amygdala. Science. 2005;308(5719):245–8. https://doi.org/10.1126/science.1105636.

38. Neumann ID. Involvement of the brain oxytocin system in stress coping: interactions with the hypothalamo-pituitary-adrenal axis. Prog Brain Res. 2002;139:147–62. https://doi.org/10.1016/S0079-6123(02)39014-9.
39. Parker KJ, Buckmaster CL, Schatzberg AF, Lyons DM. Intranasal oxytocin administration attenuates the ACTH stress response in monkeys. Psychoneuroendocrinology. 2005;30(9):924–9. https://doi.org/10.1016/j.psyneuen.2005.04.002.
40. Heinrichs M, Baumgartner T, Kirschbaum C, Ehlert U. Social support and oxytocin interact to suppress cortisol and subjective responses to psychosocial stress. Biol Psychiatry. 2003;54(12):1389–98. https://doi.org/10.1016/S0006-3223(03)00465-7.
41. de Goeij DC, Kvetnansky R, Whitnall MH, Jezova D, Berkenbosch F, Tilders FJ. Repeated stress-induced activation of corticotropin-releasing factor neurons enhances vasopressin stores and colocalization with corticotropin-releasing factor in the median eminence of rats. Neuroendocrinology. 1991;53(2):150–9. https://doi.org/10.1159/000125712.
42. Rivier C, Vale W. Modulation of stress-induced ACTH release by corticotropin-releasing factor, catecholamines and vasopressin. Nature. 1983;305(5932):325–7. https://doi.org/10.1038/305325a0.
43. Scott LV, Dinan TG. Vasopressin and the regulation of hypothalamic-pituitary-adrenal axis function: implications for the pathophysiology of depression. Life Sci. 1998;62(22):1985–98. https://doi.org/10.1016/S0024-3205(98)00027-7.
44. Larkin GL, Claassen CA, Emond JA, et al. Trends in U.S. emergency department visits for mental health conditions, 1992 to 2001. Psychiatr Serv. 2005;56:671–7.
45. Nordstrom K, Allen MH. Managing the acutely agitated and psychotic patient. CNS Spectr. 2007;12:5–11.
46. Nicolò G, Pompili E, Silvestrini C, Lagrotteria B, Laglia C. Gestione dell'aggressività cap. XIV. In: Manuale di psichiatria territoriale. Pisa: Pacini Editore Medicina; 2015.

Rapid Tranquillisation

6

Alexia E. Koukopoulos, Lavinia De Chiara,
and Georgios D. Kotzalidis

6.1 Introduction and Overview

Rapid tranquillisation refers to a drug treatment intended to calm down an individual who is supposed to suffer from agitation within a reasonably short time interval. Agitation may be reported by the patient or grossly observable by clinicians (and objectiveness here might be an issue), mainly based on observing activity, which is then compared to a culturally determined range. On one end of the continuum of motor behavioural expression is the extreme sedation and non-response to external stimuli; on the other extreme, there is extreme, uncontrolled agitation that can be assessed through specific rating scales.

Agitation may occur in a normal individual due to the acute impact of life events, especially if perceived as life-threatening and impossible to address in the specific condition in which the individual is found in that moment, or be associated with several psychiatric conditions, including schizophrenia, bipolar disorder, personality disorders (mainly antisocial and borderline personality), anxiety disorders (mostly generalised anxiety and panic), and major depressive disorder [1–6], as well as with substance use and/or intoxication [1, 7–9] or the dementias [10–15]; these conditions may affect the expression of each other [16–20]. Furthermore, agitation may be the principal clinical expression of several organic conditions due to central nervous system diseases, including Parkinson's disease, Alzheimer's disease, other types of dementia, encephalitis, meningitis and other infections, and autoimmunity [1], and of a range of systemic medical (e.g. thyrotoxicosis and hypoglycaemia) and surgical conditions, like brain traumas [1, 21].

A. E. Koukopoulos (✉)
Azienda Ospedaliera Universitaria Policlinico Umberto I, Department of Human Neurosciences, Sapienza University, Rome, Italy

L. De Chiara · G. D. Kotzalidis
UOC Psichiatria, Department of Neurosciences, Mental Health, and Sensory Organs (NESMOS), Sant'Andrea University Hospital, Sapienza University, Rome, Italy

© Springer Nature Switzerland AG 2021 93
M. Biondi et al. (eds.), *Empathy, Normalization and De-escalation*,
https://doi.org/10.1007/978-3-030-65106-0_6

When non-pharmacological interventions fail to achieve calmness, psychiatrists or other physicians have to consider pharmacological interventions, often termed "rapid tranquillisation" [22].

Agitated behaviour is associated with serious problems and challenges warranting rapid intervention, as it harbours many actual dangers for the individual involved. Indeed, it can be very stressful and may become life-threatening due to physical exhaustion and/or maladroit attempts at containment by others. Next, agitated behaviour may threaten the safety of other persons, whether family members or medical staff. Finally, it complicates the assessment and evaluation of the underlying somatic and psychiatric problems or disease.

In discussing rapid tranquillisation, the focus is always on speed, effectiveness, and safety. The context will define whether reaching calmness the soonest should prevail over obtaining patient's cooperation in deciding the best strategy to reach calmness. In cases seen at an emergency department, the context requires a prompt intravenous (IV) intervention, as safety is more frequently in jeopardy [23, 24]. Given the risk of respiratory adverse effects, the only place where performing an IV injection is safe is the emergency department, where the required specific monitoring of physical parameters is made possible. Midazolam or droperidol plus midazolam are among the best options since they allow to reach sedation in a matter of few minutes. Among the options available at an emergency department, where rapid tranquillisation is performed, IV injections act faster than intramuscular (IM) ones, and both beat in speed the oral route [23]. Oral medication is slowest in reducing agitated behaviour but preferred in contexts where collaboration is important and safety may be guaranteed through other available interventions [25]. Other alternatives consist in the intranasal and sublingual routes, and both outperform the canonical pill intake. However, most controlled studies used the IM route as a comparison. Randomised controlled trials (RCTs) studying the effects of oral medication have been studied in only six studies, which all involved risperidone [26–31]. Several consensus documents advocate oral medication or, if not otherwise possible, IM [25, 32–34]. However, most studies neglect this suggestion and use the IM route [25, 33, 35, 36]. In clinical practice, oral medication intake is preferred for practical reasons as the patient is able to self-administer the medication, thus reinforcing his/her feelings of control, mastery, and autonomy, hence potentially improving patient-staff collaboration. So, these advantages need to be balanced against the possible delay in reaching calmness using oral administration.

Guidelines advocate the use of second-generation antipsychotics [25, 32–34], but in spite of it, doctors preferably use the older antipsychotics or benzodiazepines [37, 38]. Not all second-generation antipsychotics have been tested for rapid tranquillisation or as anti-agitation agents; clozapine is not used due to its many potentially fatal side effects, but the similarly structured dibenzoazepines, olanzapine, and loxapine are currently used, as well as the piperidinic, benzisoxazole, and risperidone, but not paliperidone. Some look-warm evidence has been gathered for aripiprazole and ziprasidone, while evidence for the use of lurasidone, asenapine, brexpiprazole, and pimavanserin is only indicative and largely reserved for Alzheimer's disease patients with agitation, while for cariprazine, there are no data

pointing anywhere in agitation [39–41]; more consistent is the evidence for asenapine, which is administered sublingually [42–45]. Most guidelines or reviews are
only descriptive and offer an overview of the opportunities of pharmacological
interventions [25, 31, 36, 46, 47]. Apparently, clinicians rely heavily on clinical
experience-based evidence rather than thorough clinical studies. The level of
evidence-based on the Cochrane reviews is rather low (as usually concluded by such
reviews on any clinical issue). Studies usually focus on adult violent, aggressive, or
agitated patients, with or without specified psychopathological conditions. Special
populations, like children/adolescents or elderly people, are little investigated.
Children might need rapid tranquillisation when they develop paradoxical behavioural activation following benzodiazepine premedication prior to surgery, but their
treatment does not follow adult rules [48]. Also, studies focusing on elderly patients
are few, centred on either schizophrenia [49] or dementia [50]; however, the latter
included patients in the 55–64 year range without specifically reporting on the ≥65-
year population; other studies of acutely agitated patients included aged patients
without providing separate data for this population, one carried out in patients with
bipolar mania [51], another in patients with schizophrenia [52], and two in patients
with acute agitation and unspecified underlying disorder [53, 54]. Agitated behaviour in advanced age is frequent and difficult to handle, due to the frailty of this
population. For most antipsychotic drugs, a warning has been issued that they could
be associated with increased stroke and death rate, so clinicians now use them with
extreme caution, even at low doses.

6.2   Aims of Rapid Tranquillisation

According to the UK National Healthcare System guidelines [33, 55], rapid tranquillisation aims to calm severely agitated patients quickly, so to reduce the risk of
imminent and serious violence to self or others; rapid tranquillisation does not aim
to treat the underlying psychiatric condition, although it is recognised that improving it may reduce agitation. Rapid tranquillisation seeks not to induce sleep or
unconsciousness, nor sedation proximal to lethargy, since ideally the patient should
still be able to participate in further assessment (e.g. providing useful historical elements) and treatment decisions (consent to treatment). Hence, rapid tranquillisation
is set to procure mild sedation, which per se initiates the process of setting off
agitation.

Primary goals of all interventions aimed at treating agitated behaviour are to
ensure safety; to enhance the evaluation of underlying problems, either physical or
psychological; and to prevent further escalation; this may be reached only through
achieving calmness, as opposed to sedation, and cooperativeness. Interventions are
aimed at benefitting primarily the patient and secondarily the environment (other
people or property).

Acute pharmacological interventions aim to reach calmness and cooperativeness
within a short timeframe of maximum 2 h (arbitrarily set).

6.3   General Principles to Follow When Treating an Agitated Patient

After assessing patients' capacity to consent to treatment and risk of taking vs. risk of not taking acutely approved (off-label treatment is recommended against) medications and found that the latter outweighs the former, patients should be put in the condition that enables them to received treatment. This is to mean that both action and the lack of it should be weighed against an established benefit-to-risk ratio. Medications used in rapid tranquillisation include antipsychotics and benzodiazepines, but anti-H1 antihistamines may be associated with the former, as they sedate and induce somnolence (which are not the aims of rapid tranquillisation, but sometimes doctors cannot do without). When using sleep inducers, it is difficult to separate calmness from somnolence, but this could be an acceptable price to pay in cases of extreme agitation. Among the antipsychotics, the so-called "second-generation" drugs are preferred by consensus guidelines, but not by clinicians, a fact that casts a shadow on how "evidence" is obtained (or mongered).

When deciding which medication to use, clinicians should take into account:

- Patient's service and treatment preferences (not if against patient's interest themselves)
- Statements and decisions the patient had made in advance (including biologic testament)
- Pre-existing physical health problems
- Possible intoxication (alcohol intoxication is frequent; beware of the use of novel psychoactive substances)
- Previous response to medications to be used, including adverse events
- Potential for interactions with other drugs

When elderly people with cognitive impairment are agitated, non-pharmacological means should be preferred, as the usual drugs used in rapid tranquillisation are likely to increase acutely their probability to undergo cerebrovascular accidents [56, 57], but also because their comparative efficacy is questionable [58]. Alternative programmes for their treatment are available [14, 59, 60] and should be tried first.

6.4   Assessment. Aetiology and Differential Diagnosis

The assessment of an agitated patient is complicated by several difficulties. Uncooperativeness and/or inability to provide a reliable history often leaves clinicians in an uncomfortable situation to need to make decisions based on very limited information and under time pressure. Usually, a reliable psychiatric assessment should await that the patient is calm enough and in control to engage in a psychiatric interview [61]. The administration of standardised psychiatric interviews and clinician-rated and self-rating scales during agitation may further irritate the patient and exacerbate it, with the potential risk of a rapid escalation from agitation to aggressiveness or violence, self-directed or against others (staff or accompanying relatives and friends). Such actions are not part of the agitation per se but may constitute its complications [62]. The escalation from anxiety to agitated and violent behaviours may often be quite unpredictable, especially if the patient is unknown to the staff of the service to which he/she refers or if he/she refers to that service for the first time [63]. In these cases, the presence of clinicians who have in the past visited the patient and have gained his/her trust could be helpful to avoid all those errors that could lead to escalation and reduce unpredictability but is not often available.

One of the most dreaded sequels of agitation is suicidal acts, impulsively, but sometimes successfully, carried out [64–70]. Suicide risk is the first measure to assess in contexts of agitation and threatening behaviour; clinicians should not underestimate its importance, also because it is laid with forensic and legal complications [71].

During agitation, the assessment process should be considerably hastened. Clinicians should initially assess quickly patient's mental status, pointing to identify the most likely causes of agitation. This will provide the clinician with sufficient information to opt for initial non-pharmacological interventions to calm down the patient without sedating him/her. Once the goal is obtained, a detailed psychiatric assessment may be made possible. Diagnosis at this stage is not the primary goal, as the aim is to render the patient accessible to interview and communication. The possible value of differential diagnosis at this stage relies on allowing the clinician to avoid possible erroneous rapid tranquillisation approaches. For example, in the case of an elderly man with agitation whose main diagnosis is unknown, it is important to assess recent drug intake history, accidental or not, so to rule out possible paradoxical reactions to benzodiazepines, in which case further benzodiazepine or antipsychotic drug administration could prove to be useless or even perilous. Differential diagnosis at this stage should be directed at safety issues, so to develop an appropriate treatment strategy [61]. Agitation could be the end result of processes of different aetiologies, either medical or psychiatric [31, 72]. This is the reason why agitation is one of the most common clinical problems in psychiatric facilities and emergency services [31].

To establish the best treatment strategy at a state of agitation of unknown origin, it is important that an immediate underlying cause of the agitation is tentatively established. An expert consensus identified three general possible aetiologies of agitation, i.e. a general medical condition, substance intoxication, and a primary psychiatric disorder [73], with a fourth category of undifferentiated agitation added by the BETA project workgroup [61, 72]. In contrast, the Austrian guidelines [32] proposed a detailed classification which included catatonic, manic, and agitated depressive syndromes, disturbance of consciousness/delirium, suicidality, delusions, hallucinations, anxiety/panic syndromes, alcohol and/or drug use, and dementia. This classification requires an expert clinician to deal with agitation.

The initial differential diagnosis, albeit imprecise as to the biological underpinnings of agitation, is necessary for adopting adequate treatment strategies. At this stage, rather than targeting the right treatment, it is essential to select the treatment that will address the situation while avoiding errors that could worsen the short-term prognosis.

6.5   Assessing Agitated Behaviour

Although there are several scales assessing objectively the severity of agitation, like the Overt Agitation Severity Scale [74], the Stanford Scale for Agitation Symptoms [75], and the New Hamburg-Hannover Agitation Scale [76], they have not achieved wide diffusion in rapid tranquillisation contexts. The most frequently used primary outcomes in such contexts are the scores obtained on the PANSS-EC at the second hour post-injection. The PANSS-EC is the Excited Component of the Positive and Negative Syndrome Scale (PANSS) [77] and consists of the following PANSS items: P4, Excitement; G14, Poor impulse control; G4, Tension; P7, Hostility; and G8, Uncooperativeness. Each item is rated for severity on a Likert scale ranging from 1 (absent) to 7 (extreme).

The most used secondary outcome is the score on the Agitation-Calmness Evaluation Scale (ACES) [78], a single-item, 9-point Likert scale where 1 is marked agitation, 2 moderate agitation, 3 mild agitation, 4 normal, 5 mild calmness, 6 moderate calmness, 7 calmness, 8 deep sleep, and 9 unarousable (optimum is a score in the 4–8 range, while 9 is oversedation, a side effect).

ACES and PEC should be administered to evaluate psychomotor agitation/ excitement 30, 60, 90, and 120 min following drug administration; measurements should be repeated 24 h later. The PANSS-EC score is used to determine whether the administration of the drug should be repeated; if it does not show a reduction of a least 40%, the dose has to be repeated. In case of lack of improvement or recurrence 2 h after administration, dosing is repeated and the patient re-evaluated after further 2 h and so on. Meanwhile, the clinicians attempt at getting in touch with the patient, so to de-escalate aggressiveness and avoid escalating with drug dose.

Response is usually judged according to the scores on the PANSS-EC and ACES; non-response is considered 5 on the PANSS-EC and 1 on the ACES, low response is 4 on the PANSS-EC and 2 on the ACES, fair response is 2–3 on the PANSS-EC and 3 on the ACES, and remission is 1 on the PANSS-EC and 4 on the ACES; with no symptoms at all, the patient is considered to have completely recovered.

6.6   Reduced Agitated Behaviour
and Meta-analytic Findings

Lorazepam was found to reduce the PANSS-EC by at least 7 points in a meta-analysis [23]. Haloperidol was found to reduce it by 7–8 points, while its combination with promethazine has been assessed in only one study but showed an impressive reduction by 15 points after 2 h. In contrast, the combination of haloperidol plus lorazepam showed more consistently a less strong reduction, i.e. by 8–10 points after 2 h. Finally, the combination of haloperidol with midazolam resulted in a 15-point PANSS-EC score reduction after only 90 min in one study. We could presume that study similarity or remakes ensue in a reduction of effect sizes.

Levomepromazine has been used in two studies in a more elderly population, resulting in a decrease of 5–6 PANSS-EC points. Aripiprazole usually reduces

PANSS-EC scores between 7 and 8 points save for one study, which found a reduction of only 3 points [79]. Cumulative evidence is low quality for IM aripiprazole and indicates a small effect size, as it emerges from a Cochrane review [80], but strict inclusion criteria adopted by these reviews are likely to result in few studies meeting the criteria and the consequent complaint of poor quality of evidence and the need for further studies.

Olanzapine showed a decrease around 7–10 points on the PANSS-EC. Two hours following acute administration, risperidone reduced scores on the PANSS-EC by 7–8 points in two studies [29, 30] and by 14 points in one [81].

Adding lorazepam or clonazepam to risperidone does not achieve a further decrease on the PANSS-EC score [29]. Ziprasidone reduced PANSS-EC score by 3–15. Loxapine, which is currently used as nasal inhalation, results in 9–11 point reduction. Finally, placebo also showed a 2–6 point reduction after 2 h on the PANSS-EC [23].

Summarising, risperidone shows the most robust change of >14 points on the PANSS-EC after 2 h; it is followed by olanzapine, aripiprazole, and haloperidol plus lorazepam. The administration of any of these drugs resulted in a decrease on the PANSS-EC of more than 8 points at the 2-h time point [23].

Risperidone combined with lorazepam, lorazepam alone, risperidone combined with clonazepam, and haloperidol alone were followed 2 h later by modest decreases in agitation (a 6–8-point decrease on the PANSS-EC). Levomepromazine, ziprasidone, and placebo hardly showed any clinically relevant decrease of agitated behaviour.

6.7   Proportion of Patients Reaching Calmness

6.7.1   Benzodiazepines

With lorazepam, 63–88% of patients are calm 120 min after medication. About 78% reaches calmness within 15–20 min. With midazolam, only one study reported that 95% of patients reached calmness after 120 min [82], whereas 55–89% of them had reached calmness already within 15–20 min.

6.7.2   Antipsychotics (With or Without Additional Medication)

Two hours after haloperidol administration, 60–89% of patients reach calmness [83–85]. A similar proportion of patients (55–92%) successfully reaches calmness even in the shorter term (15–20 min) [84].

With the haloperidol plus promethazine combination, 67–91% of patients achieve calmness within 15–20 min; this increases to 89–97% 2 h after administration. With droperidol, 53–92% of patients reaches calmness within 15–20 min and 96% after 60 min [86]. Combining droperidol with IV midazolam, 89% of patients reached calmness within 15–20 min and 98% after 60 min [87].

As for second-generation antipsychotic drugs, olanzapine resulted in calmness in 73–91% of agitated patients after 2 h, with 66% reaching it already after 15–20 min if administered IV. Two hours after aripiprazole administration, 60–84% of the patients achieved calmness; this was 29–90% for ziprasidone, 66–74% for loxapine (which is not strictly a second-generation antipsychotic drug and found currently use as intranasal spray), and 28–44% for placebo [23].

Taken together, these fragmentary data point to rapid tranquillisation reaching calmness in a considerable proportion of agitated patients in a matter of 15–20 min, but most of those who resist finally yield after about 2 h. However, a small percentage of patients takes longer to respond or do not respond at all.

6.8   Time Needed to Reach Calmness

The time needed to obtain calmness is an individually important measure but quite unimportant considering an agitated population and the wide standard deviation expected. In fact, inter- and intraindividual factors may affect it, and it is not definable even in the same patient on the basis of drug intake history, which is however important for clinical decisions. However, some studies reported for statistical completeness the mean time in minutes that patients needed to reach calmness [23].

The usual route of administration route is IM, as oral administration may not always be possible due to the fact that most patients are uncooperative and resist taking medication and have to be treated in a compulsory regimen. Other administration routes are by inhalation, with loxapine the only available agent, which reaches calmness in 2–67 min [23, 88, 89], while IV administration has been used only in one study reporting time to calmness [87]. This study compared IV droperidol 10 mg with IV olanzapine 10 mg and IV midazolam 5 mg plus droperidol 5 mg and found that by reducing droperidol to half its dose and adding the benzodiazepine, the time to calmness could be extremely shortened compared to the two antipsychotics alone. The median time to calmness was 5 min (range 3–11) with the droperidol-midazolam combination, outperforming antipsychotics alone (median time to calmness 11 min for both droperidol and olanzapine, ranges 6–23 and 5–25, respectively) [87]. The only study assessing oral administration compared 2 mg oral liquid risperidone plus 2 mg oral lorazepam with 5 mg IM haloperidol plus 2 mg IM lorazepam [26]. In this study, all patients were sleeping within 45 min, with no between-groups differences.

Median time to sedation for individual antipsychotics administered alone was 30 min for haloperidol, 11–20 min for droperidol, and 11–30 for olanzapine [23, 87, 90]. Adding the antihistaminic promethazine to haloperidol barely improves the above figure (20–30 min). Combining haloperidol with midazolam considerably accelerates the achievement of calmness (about 10 min) but does not allow to reduce the dosage, as in the case of droperidol plus lorazepam, which permits to reduce to 2.5 mg the IM antipsychotic and achieves calmness in 15 min, while lorazepam alone achieves it in 40 min [90].

Regarding benzodiazepines alone, lorazepam was associated in one study with reaching calmness in a mean of 48 min and midazolam in 20–24 min. It should be recalled that midazolam has anaesthetic properties, while lorazepam is devoid of such actions.

No data are available for other drugs used in rapid tranquillisation or placebo [23].

Summarising, antipsychotics and benzodiazepines or antihistaminic drugs (major and minor tranquillisers, respectively) are the mainstay of rapid tranquillisation; although it is safer to start with a minor tranquilliser if the patient's basic condition is unknown, combining the two speeds up the process of sedation.

6.9   Adverse Events

During rapid tranquillisation, the adverse events that are usually related to the use of the employed drugs are fewer, due to the limited time of tranquillising treatment exposure, but when they occur, they may be abrupt and life-threatening and have to be addressed in an emergency context. Both major drug classes used in rapid tranquillisation, i.e. antipsychotics and benzodiazepines, due to their sleep-facilitating properties, which is part of the tranquillisation process, may affect alertness and movement. Antipsychotics are likely to be related to sedation due to their H1 antihistaminic properties, but not all antipsychotics share these properties. Phenothiazines like chlorpromazine and levomepromazine are potent antihistaminics, while butyrophenones like haloperidol and droperidol do little on histamine receptors. Benzodiazepines, on the other hand, facilitate GABA binding on the $GABA_A$ receptors, thus inducing relaxation. With concurrent antipsychotic-benzodiazepine administration, which is becoming the rule in rapid tranquillisation of the severely agitated patient, it is possible that an interplay between these mechanisms could lead to oversedation. The picture is further complicated by the fact that any intervention has a placebo component, which is mainly consisting of patient's, doctor's, and social expectations that may reinforce sedative effects.

6.9.1   Oversedation

The extent to which medications are related with oversedation varies. The figures reported are 10% for lorazepam, 0–36% for haloperidol, paradoxically 3% for haloperidol plus promethazine, 13–70% for haloperidol plus lorazepam, 40% for haloperidol plus midazolam, 1% for droperidol, 4–9% for aripiprazole, 3–13% for olanzapine, 13% for risperidone, 13% for risperidone plus lorazepam, 8% for levomepromazine, 10% for ziprasidone, 11–13% for loxapine, and 2–10% placebo [23]. These figures tell us of the importance of placebo mechanisms and of the need for placebo-controlled studies when we deal with rapid tranquillisation.

6.9.2   Movement Disorders

Sedation proportionally causes slowing down of intentional motion and reduced precision in executing movements. These become increasingly sluggish due to both centrally induced and peripheral relaxation. However, there are some paradoxical reactions that may also occur during rapid tranquillisation.

6.9.2.1 Benzodiazepines
Extrapyramidal symptoms (EPS) like acute dystonia and akathisia are absent with lorazepam and midazolam, save for one study reporting 2% of akathisia for loraze-pam [23]. Summarising, acute movement disorders are not to be expected with benzodiazepines.

6.9.2.2 Antipsychotics
Haloperidol-related EPS were found in 6–55% of cases, with acute dystonia between 0% and 17% and akathisia 8–46%. Figures for haloperidol plus promethazine are unreliable, as EPS reports vary from 0% to 74%; however, no acute dystonia or akathisia have been reported [23]. For haloperidol plus lorazepam, EPS were 5% and acute dystonia 3%, while for haloperidol plus midazolam, occurrences were 44% and 10%, respectively. Droperidol, with or without midazolam, showed low movement disorder occurrences, with 0% EPS, 0–1% acute dystonia, and 0% akathisia. Aripiprazole has been associated with 2% EPS in one study, 1–2% acute dystonia, and 3% akathisia [23]. For olanzapine, these proportions were 0–5% EPS, 0–4% acute dystonia, and 0–2% akathisia and, for risperidone, 6–8% EPS and 2% acute dystonia, with no variations after adding lorazepam or clonazepam [23]. Levomepromazine has been associated with 8% akathisia, but no EPSs or acute dystonia. EPSs were reported in 52% of cases receiving ziprasidone on one study [91]. For intranasal loxapine, there are no reports of movement disorders. Finally, 2–7% EPS were reported with placebo, but no reports of acute dystonia or akathisia [23]. Taken together, these data suggest that movement disorders ought to be carefully watched during rapid tranquillisation but are not important concerns. Sometimes, acute oculogyric crises may occur that should be promptly addressed with benztropine or antihistaminic drugs.

6.9.3   Cardiovascular Adverse Effects

Sudden death due to cardiac arrest has been a major concern for classical neuroleptic drugs since the launch of second-generation antipsychotics. This was followed by the withdrawal from the market of thioridazine and the progressive drop of the use of haloperidol. Economic reasons related to industrial policies may lie behind this. QTc prolongation, which is defined as QTc time >450 ms, may increase the risk of arrhythmias, thus exposing the patient to the risk of cardiac arrest. QTc prolongation is a common feature of older antipsychotics; however, second-generation antipsychotics are not free from this dreaded side effect [34, 55].

6.9.3.1 Benzodiazepines

QTc prolongation is quite rare with benzodiazepine treatment and more so during the short time of rapid tranquillisation. One study comparing aripiprazole with lorazepam in rapid tranquillisation reported QTc prolongation in 4% of cases treated with aripiprazole and 7% of lorazepam [92]. For midazolam, 3–7% of cases in rapid tranquillisation were found to be associated with QTc prolongation [23].

6.9.3.2 Antipsychotics

QTc prolongation is an issue with prolonged antipsychotic treatment but may also arise in acute treatment, such as that of rapid tranquillisation. In rapid tranquillisation studies, haloperidol has been associated with QTc prolongation in 0–6% of cases, droperidol alone in 1–6%, combined with midazolam in 1–14%, aripiprazole in 0–6% (not related to dose), and olanzapine in 0–3%. Placebo was associated with QT prolongation in 2.4–8% of cases [23, 92, 93]. Electrocardiographic monitoring is recommended during rapid tranquillisation, although QTc > 450 ms is an infrequent finding.

6.9.4 Alterations in Blood Pressure

Hypertension is an issue for some antipsychotic drugs, like olanzapine and levomepromazine [23]. Their effects on biogenic amines might underlie the triggering of hypertensive crises that could be extremely dangerous in contexts of agitation and rapid tranquillisation. Blood pressure should always be monitored during rapid tranquillisation, despite patient's uncooperativeness.

Hypotension with antipsychotics could also be due to biogenic amine interactions and their antidopaminergic effects on heart dopamine receptors. Hypotension is a more frequent problem with antipsychotics than hypertension. Hypertension was found in 3% of cases treated with levomepromazine, while hypotension was found in 16% of patients. Hypotension is more likely with benzodiazepines because they act on peripheral receptors that relax arterioles. However, clinically relevant hypotension in rapid tranquillisation settings was 5% with midazolam, while figures for haloperidol varied from 0% to 17% when given alone, 10% when associated with promethazine, 3% when combined with lorazepam, and 10% when combined with midazolam. With droperidol, the occurrence of hypotension is low, 0–4%, but with the droperidol-midazolam combination, this rises to 2–41%. Hypotension with olanzapine occurs in 0–4% of cases [23].

6.9.5 Hypoventilation and Respiratory Depression

This is a rare problem for antipsychotics and a frequent one for benzodiazepines. These drugs tend to depress the medullary respiratory centres through GABAergic mechanisms [94]; hence, treating physicians must ensure the availability of the

GABA$_A$ receptor antagonist flumazenil as a life-saving medication. In rapid tranquillisation contexts, midazolam was shown to be associated with increased saturation problems, especially in patients with ethanol intoxication. Ventilatory support should be available for these cases.

6.9.6   Throat Irritation

Sore throat (1–7%) and dysgeusia (4–17%) are shown only with loxapine, presumably because of its intranasal formulation.

What Does the Doctor Need When Performing Rapid Tranquillisation?
Rapid tranquillisation is an act of great responsibility since, in many instances, agitated patients refuse treatment. The first concern of the physician should be to assess the patient's capacity to consent to treatment. Not assessing it might expose the physician to legal repercussions. Patients whose agitation is rooted in an anxiety, post-traumatic, or depressive disorder are likely to be capable to express consent to treatment and do not pose particular problems to the clinician; they are also likely to accept oral treatment, and the only threat comes from their movements, which may be brisk, precipitous, unadvised, and unpredictable. However, some patients may be capable to express consent, and they refuse to accept treatment. These patients should not be treated. For patients who cannot express valid consent to treatment, they may be treated under compulsory regimen. When rapid tranquillisation is decided, the clinician must have at hand data on vital signs, i.e. blood pressure, pulse and heart rate, temperature, respiratory rate, hydration, blood oxygen saturation (to measure with pulse oximeters), level of consciousness, and any side effects; all the above must be monitored and recorded on the patient's clinical record at close intervals (5–10 min if possible). If the patient refuses monitoring, at least respiratory rate, mucosal hydration and level of consciousness must be annotated [55]. The equipment that should be available in every rapid tranquillisation context includes pulse oximeters, electrocardiographs, oxygen supply, and defibrillator. Resuscitation drugs should also be available (opioid and GABA antagonists, beta-adrenoceptor agonists, noradrenaline).

When an agitated patient is not collaborative and is incapacitated to provide valid consent for treatment, he/she may be treated compulsorily. The patient may be put in physical restraint to allow rapid tranquillisation to take place. Restrictive interventions, physical or mechanical restraint, are traditionally used for managing disruptive/violent behaviours in psychiatry [95]. One of the restrictive measures involves seclusion in a safe, bare room with soft walls and floor, to avoid that the patient could hurt him/herself [96], but such room is not available in all services and in all countries.

6.10   Suggestions from Treatment Guidelines and Clinical Experience

Combining the evidence discussed by consensus papers and treatment guidelines, several recommendations may be made. Haloperidol should not be used IV as it has obtained no clear evidence of utility in rapid tranquillisation [89]. Promethazine should never be combined with lorazepam [55]. If a patient is amidst an alcoholic intoxication, avoid benzodiazepines, as they may potentiate the effects of ethanol in the brain and worsen effects of haloperidol [97]. Do not administer benzodiazepines in patients who are long-term benzodiazepine users. The odds that a patient will promptly respond to promethazine alone are high, so it is better to start with this drug and possibly add haloperidol after the patient showed non-response. Do not use haloperidol in patients with cardiovascular disease and benzodiazepines in patients with respiratory problems.

Patients of paediatric age should not be treated with rapid tranquillisation, as there are no standards applying to this patient population. Adult patients (18–65 years of age) should receive a first proposal for oral therapy, and if they accept, 1–2 mg lorazepam should be administered as first line (maximum, 4 mg/day). Alternatively, they may receive haloperidol 5–10 mg (maximum 20 mg/day). As second-line treatment, they may receive risperidone (1–2 mg, maximum daily 4 mg) or olanzapine (5–10 mg, maximum daily 20 mg), or promethazine alone (25 mg, and if needed, another 25 mg dose, with no further repeat, or 50 mg in one shot and no more promethazine for the whole day) or with haloperidol. Repeat administration should be carried out at 45 min intervals.

Adult patients refusing oral medication should be treated with 2 mg IM lorazepam that may be repeated just once in that day [33]. Otherwise, they may receive haloperidol 5 mg (maximum daily 20 mg) plus promethazine 25–50 mg (maximum daily 100 mg) [33], or promethazine alone at the same doses. When the risk of EPSs is established, aripiprazole 9.75 mg (maximum 30 mg/day) with lorazepam 2 mg (maximum 4 mg/day), or aripiprazole alone, is to be repeated after 2 h in case of partial response.

For the elderly patient, the general approach is similar, but the doses are reduced to about half, save for aripiprazole.

The bioavailability and peak concentrations of benzodiazepines do not differ much between oral and IM administration, while for antipsychotics, they are respectively considerably increased and shortened with the IM administration. IV administration shortens plasma peak extremely but is not much used in rapid tranquillisation.

Although the *Maudsley Prescribing Guidelines* [34] support the use of droperidol in rapid tranquillisation, NICE-NHS-related [33, 55] and the Österreichische Gesellschaft für Neuropsychopharmakologie und Biologische Psychiatrie [32] guidelines do not provide for the use of droperidol, which has the potential to increase QTc interval like haloperidol, but fared as one of the best options, especially when combined with benzodiazepines, according to the evidence provided above. However, an updated Cochrane review found it to be effective for the treatment of acutely agitated patients and no evidence to suggest that it should not be used in such context [98]. Its use with a benzodiazepine to be as effective as olanzapine [99]. Droperidol is a difficult to manage medication and should be administered in controlled, hospital settings, but data so far indicate its place in rapid tranquillisation should be reconsidered.

6.11   Conclusions

Rapid tranquillisation is aimed at reaching calmness and restoring normal contact with one's own environment as soon as possible. The effect of tranquillising medication is controlled every 20–30 min with oral formulations, every 5–10 min with IM or IV formulations, and every 2–20 min with inhaled loxapine. If the patient has not improved in 30–60 min, a repeat dose may be administered. The tranquillisation process is expected to be complete within 2 h. If agitation persists for more than 2 h, repeat doses may be given being careful not to overcome the maximum allowed dose for each drug. The use of a given drug depends not only on past clinical evidence but also on availability in the structure where the treating physician is called to administer rapid tranquillisation (hospital or clinic pharmacies).

References

1. Battaglia J. Pharmacological management of acute agitation. Drugs. 2005;65(9):1207–22. https://doi.org/10.2165/00003495-200565090-00003.
2. Fountoulakis KN, Leucht S, Kaprinis GS. Personality disorders and violence. Curr Opin Psychiatry. 2008;21(1):84–92. https://doi.org/10.1097/YCO.0b013e3282f31137.
3. Hassanzadah M, Bitar AH, Khanfar NM, Khasawneh FT, Lutfy K, Shankar GS. A retrospective cohort study of the prevalence of anxiety and agitation in schizophrenic smokers and the unmet needs of smoking cessation programs. Medicine. 2019;98(40):e17375. https://doi.org/10.1097/MD.0000000000017375.
4. Nordstrom K, Allen MH. Managing the acutely agitated and psychotic patient. CNS Spectr. 2007;12(10 Suppl 17):5–11. https://doi.org/10.1017/s1092852900026286.
5. Roberts J, Gracia Canales A, Blanthorn-Hazell S, Craciun Boldeanu A, Judge D. Characterizing the experience of agitation in patients with bipolar disorder and schizophrenia. BMC Psychiatry. 2018;18(1):104. https://doi.org/10.1186/s12888-018-1673-3.
6. Sacchetti E, Valsecchi P, Tamussi E, Paulli L, Morigi R, Vita A. Psychomotor agitation in subjects hospitalized for an acute exacerbation of Schizophrenia. Psychiatry Res. 2018;270:357–64. https://doi.org/10.1016/j.psychres.2018.09.058.
7. Citrome L. New treatments for agitation. Psychiatry Q. 2004;75(3):197–213. https://doi.org/10.1023/b:psaq.0000031791.53142.85.
8. Cole JB, Klein LR, Martel ML. Parenteral antipsychotic choice and its association with emergency department length of stay for acute agitation secondary to alcohol intoxication. Acad Emerg Med. 2019;26(1):79–84. https://doi.org/10.1111/acem.13486.
9. Pepa PA, Lee KC, Huynh HE, Wilson MP. Safety of risperidone for acute agitation and alcohol intoxication in Emergency Department patients. J Emerg Med. 2017;53(4):530–5. https://doi.org/10.1016/j.jemermed.2017.05.028.

10. Anatchkova M, Brooks A, Swett L, Hartry A, Duffy RA, Baker RA, Hammer-Helmich L, Sanon AM. Agitation in patients with dementia: a systematic review of epidemiology and association with severity and course. Int Psychogeriatr. 2019;31:1305–18. https://doi.org/10.1017/S1041610218001898.

11. Ijaopo EO. Dementia-related agitation: a review of non-pharmacological interventions and analysis of risks and benefits of pharmacotherapy. Transl Psychiatry. 2017;7(10):e1250. https://doi.org/10.1038/tp.2017.199.

12. Keszycki RM, Fisher DW, Dong H. The hyperactivity-impulsivity-irritiability-disinhibition-aggression-agitation domain in Alzheimer's disease: current management and future directions. Front Pharmacol. 2019;10:1109. https://doi.org/10.3389/fphar.2019.01109.

13. Liu KY, Stringer AE, Reeves SJ, Howard RJ. The neurochemistry of agitation in Alzheimer's disease: a systematic review. Ageing Res Rev. 2018;43:99–107. https://doi.org/10.1016/j.arr.2018.03.003.

14. Marston L, Livingston G, Laybourne A, Cooper C. Becoming or remaining agitated: the course of agitation in people with dementia living in care homes. The English Longitudinal Managing Agitation and Raising Quality of Life (MARQUE) study. J Alzheimers Dis. 2020;76(2):467–73. https://doi.org/10.3233/JAD-191195.

15. Rosenberg PB, Wanigatunga SK, Spira AP. The potential of actigraphy to assess agitation in dementia. Am J Geriatr Psychiatry. 2019;27(8):870–2. https://doi.org/10.1016/j.jagp.2019.03.009.

16. Angst J, Gamma A, Benazzi F, Ajdacic V, Rössler W. Does psychomotor agitation in major depressive episodes indicate bipolarity? Evidence from the Zurich Study. Eur Arch Psychiatry Clin Neurosci. 2009;259(1):55–63. https://doi.org/10.1007/s00406-008-0834-7.

17. Bassir Nia A, Mann CL, Spriggs S, DeFrancisco DR, Carbonaro S, Parvez L, Galynker II, Perkel CA, Hurd YL. The relevance of sex in the association of synthetic cannabinoid use with psychosis and agitation in an inpatient population. J Clin Psychiatry. 2019;80(4):18m12539. https://doi.org/10.4088/JCP.18m12539.

18. Leventhal AM, Zimmerman M. The relative roles of bipolar disorder and psychomotor agitation in substance dependence. Psychol Addict Behav. 2010;24(2):360–5. https://doi.org/10.1037/a0019217.

19. Mintzer JE, Brawman-Mintzer O. Agitation as a possible expression of generalized anxiety disorder in demented elderly patients: toward a treatment approach. J Clin Psychiatry. 1996;57(Suppl 7):55–63; discussion 73–5

20. Ruthirakuhan M, Lanctôt KL, Vieira D, Herrmann N. Natural and synthetic cannabinoids for agitation and aggression in Alzheimer's disease: a meta-analysis. J Clin Psychiatry. 2019;80(2):18r12617. https://doi.org/10.4088/JCP.18r12617.

21. Warren RE, Deary IJ, Frier BM. The symptoms of hyperglycaemia in people with insulin-treated diabetes: classification using principal components analysis. Diabetes Metab Res Rev. 2003;19(5):408–14. https://doi.org/10.1002/dmrr.396.

22. Cookson J. Rapid tranquillisation: the science and advice. BJPsych Adv. 2018;24(5):346–58. https://doi.org/10.1192/bja.2018.25.

23. Bak M, Weltens I, Bervoets C, De Fruyt J, Samochowiec J, Fiorillo A, Sampogna G, Bienkowski P, Preuss WU, Misiak B, Frydecka D, Samochowiec A, Bak E, Drukker M, Dom G. The pharmacological management of agitated and aggressive behaviour: a systematic review and meta-analysis. Eur Psychiatry. 2019;57:78–100. https://doi.org/10.1016/j.eurpsy.2019.01.014.

24. Jibson MD. Psychopharmacology in the emergency room. J Clin Psychiatry. 2007;68(5):796–7. https://doi.org/10.4088/jcp.v68n0521.

25. Garriga M, Pacchiarotti I, Kasper S, Zeller SL, Allen MH, Vázquez G, Baldaçara L, San L, McAllister-Williams RH, Fountoulakis KN, Courtet P, Naber D, Chan EW, Fagiolini A, Möller HJ, Grunze H, Llorca PM, Jaffe RL, Yatham LN, Hidalgo-Mazzei D, Passamar M, Messer T, Bernardo M, Vieta E. Assessment and management of agitation in psychiatry: expert consensus. World J Biol Psychiatry. 2016;17(2):86–128. https://doi.org/10.3109/15622975.2015.1132007.

26. Currier GW, Simpson GM. Risperidone liquid concentrate and oral lorazepam versus intramuscular haloperidol and intramuscular lorazepam for treatment of psychotic agitation. J Clin Psychiatry. 2001;62(3):153–7. https://doi.org/10.4088/jcp.v62n0303.

27. Currier GW, Chou JC, Feifel D, Bossie CA, Turkoz I, Mahmoud RA, Gharabawi GM. Acute treatment of psychotic agitation: a randomized comparison of oral treatment with risperidone and lorazepam versus intramuscular treatment with haloperidol and lorazepam. J Clin Psychiatry. 2004;65(3):386–94.

28. Fang M, Chen H, Li LH, Wu R, Li Y, Liu L, Ye M, Huang J, Zhu S, Wang G, Zhang Q, Zheng H, Zhang L, Wang B, Zhou J, Zhao JP. Comparison of risperidone oral solution and intramuscular haloperidol with the latter shifting to oral therapy for the treatment of acute agitation in patients with schizophrenia. Int Clin Psychopharmacol. 2012;27(2):107–13. https://doi.org/10.1097/YIC.0b013e32834fc431.

29. Hatta K, Kawabata T, Yoshida K, Hamakawa H, Wakejima T, Furuta K, Nakamura M, Hirata T, Usui C, Nakamura H, Sawa Y. Olanzapine orally disintegrating tablet vs. risperidone oral solution in the treatment of acutely agitated psychotic patients. Gen Hosp Psychiatry. 2008;30(4):367–71. https://doi.org/10.1016/j.genhosppsych.2008.03.004.

30. Lim HK, Kim JJ, Pae CU, Lee CU, Lee C, Paik IH. Comparison of risperidone orodispersible tablet and intramuscular haloperidol in the treatment of acute psychotic agitation: a randomized open, prospective study. Neuropsychobiology. 2010;62(2):81–6. https://doi.org/10.1159/000315437.

31. Yildiz A, Turgay A, Alpay M, Sachs GS. Observational data on the antiagitation effect of risperidone tablets in emergency settings: a preliminary report. Int J Psychiatry Clin Pract. 2003;7(3):217–21. https://doi.org/10.1080/13651500310000889.

32. Kasper S, Baranyi A, Eisenburger P, Erfurth A, Ertl M, Frey R, Hausmann A, Kapfhammer HP, Psota G, Rados C, Roitner-Vitzthum E, Sachs GM, Winkler D. Die Behandlung der Agitation beim psychiatrischen Notfall. Konsensus-Statement – State of the art 2013. CliniCum neuropsy Sonderausgabe. Vienna: Österreichische Gesellschaft für Neuropsychopharmakologie und Biologische Psychiatrie; 2013. https://oegpb.at/wp-content/uploads/2014/07/Kons_Agitation_psych_Notfall.pdf.

33. NICE. NICE-guideline [NG10]: violence and aggression. NICE-guideline: violence and aggression: short-term management in mental health, health and community settings: updated edition 28 May 2015. London: National Institute for Health and Care Excellence; 2015.

34. Taylor DM, Barnes TRE, Young AH. The Maudsley prescribing guidelines in psychiatry. 13th ed. Wiley-Blackwell: Chichester; 2018. ISBN: 978-1-119-44260-8.

35. Bak M, van Os J, Marcelis M. Acute ingrijpmedicatie; literatuuroverzicht en aanbevelingen [Rapid tranquillisation; review of the literature and recommendations]. Tijdschr Psychiatr. 2011;53(10):727–37.

36. Rocca P, Villari V, Bogetto F. Managing the aggressive and violent patient in the psychiatric emergency. Prog Neuropsychopharmacol Biol Psychiatry. 2006;30(4):586–98. https://doi.org/10.1016/j.pnpbp.2006.01.015.

37. Bervoets C, Roelant E, De Fruyt J, Demunter H, Dekeyser B, Vandenbussche L, Titeca K, Pieters G, Sabbe B, Morrens M. Prescribing preferences in rapid tranquillisation: a survey in Belgian psychiatrists and emergency physicians. BMC Res Notes. 2015;8:218. https://doi.org/10.1186/s13104-015-1172-2.

38. Wilson MP, Minassian A, Bahramzi M, Campillo A, Vilke GM. Despite expert recommendations, second-generation antipsychotics are not often prescribed in the emergency department. J Emerg Med. 2014;46(6):808–13. https://doi.org/10.1016/j.jemermed.2014.01.017.

39. Allen MH, Citrome L, Pikalov A, Hsu J, Loebel A. Efficacy of lurasidone in the treatment of agitation: a post hoc analysis of five short-term studies in acutely ill patients with schizophrenia. Gen Hosp Psychiatry. 2017;47:75–82. https://doi.org/10.1016/j.genhosppsych.2017.05.002.

40. Caraci F, Santagati M, Caruso G, Cannavò D, Leggio GM, Salomone S, Drago F. New antipsychotic drugs for the treatment of agitation and psychosis in Alzheimer's disease: focus on brexpiprazole and pimavanserin. F1000Res. 2020;9:F1000. https://doi.org/10.12688/f1000research.22662.1. Faculty Rev-686.

41. Stummer L, Markovic M, Maroney M. Brexpiprazole in the treatment of schizophrenia and agitation in Alzheimer's disease. Neurodegener Dis Manag. 2020;10(4):205–17. https://doi.org/10.2217/nmt-2020-0013.
42. Amon JS, Johnson SB, El-Mallakh RS. Asenapine for the control of physical aggression: a prospective naturalist pilot study. Psychopharmacol Bull. 2017;47(1):27–32.
43. Citrome L, Landbloom R, Chang CT, Earley W. Effects of asenapine on agitation and hostility in adults with acute manic or mixed episodes associated with bipolar I disorder. Neuropsychiatr Dis Treat. 2017;13:2955–63. https://doi.org/10.2147/NDT.S149376.
44. Pratts M, Citrome L, Grant W, Leso L, Opler LA. A single-dose, randomized, double-blind, placebo-controlled trial of sublingual asenapine for acute agitation. Acta Psychiatr Scand. 2014;130(1):61–8. https://doi.org/10.1111/acps.12262.
45. Zun LS. Evidence-based review of pharmacotherapy for acute agitation. Part 1: onset of efficacy. J Emerg Med. 2018;54(3):364–74. https://doi.org/10.1016/j.jemermed.2017.10.011.
46. Hockenhull JC, Whittington R, Leitner M, Barr W, McGuire J, Cherry MG, Flentje R, Quinn B, Dundar Y, Dickson R. A systematic review of prevention and intervention strategies for populations at high risk of engaging in violent behaviour: update 2002-8. Health Technol Assess. 2012;16(3):1–152. https://doi.org/10.3310/hta16030.
47. Pratt JP, Chandler-Oats J, Nelstrop L, Branford D, Pereira S. Establishing gold standard approaches to rapid tranquillisation: a review and discussion of the evidence on the safety and efficacy of medications currently used. J Psychiatr Intens Care. 2008;4(1&2):43–57. https://doi.org/10.1017/S1742646408001234.
48. Golparvar M, Saghaei M, Sajedi P, Razavi SS. Paradoxical reaction following intravenous midazolam premedication in pediatric patients – a randomized placebo controlled trial of ketamine for rapid tranquilization. Paediatr Anaesth. 2004;14(11):924–30. https://doi.org/10.1111/j.1460-9592.2004.01349.x.
49. Suzuki H, Gen K. A naturalistic comparison of the efficacy and safety of intramuscular olanzapine and intramuscular levomepromazine in agitated elderly patients with schizophrenia. Neuropsychiatr Dis Treat. 2013;9:1281–7. https://doi.org/10.2147/NDT.S50754.
50. Rappaport SA, Marcus RN, Manos G, McQuade RD, Oren DA. A randomized, double-blind, placebo-controlled tolerability study of intramuscular aripiprazole in acutely agitated patients with Alzheimer's, vascular, or mixed dementia. J Am Med Dir Assoc. 2009;10(1):21–7. https://doi.org/10.1016/j.jamda.2008.06.006.
51. Meehan K, Zhang F, David S, Tohen M, Janicak P, Small J, Koch M, Rizk R, Walker D, Tran P, Breier A. A double-blind, randomized comparison of the efficacy and safety of intramuscular injections of olanzapine, lorazepam, or placebo in treating acutely agitated patients diagnosed with bipolar mania. J Clin Psychopharmacol. 2001;21(4):389–97. https://doi.org/10.1097/00004714-200108000-00006.
52. Suzuki H, Gen K, Takahashi Y. A naturalistic comparison study of the efficacy and safety of intramuscular olanzapine, intramuscular haloperidol, and intramuscular levomepromazine in acute agitated patients with schizophrenia. Hum Psychopharmacol. 2014;29(1):83–8. https://doi.org/10.1002/hup.2376.
53. Dubin WR, Weiss KJ. Rapid tranquilization: a comparison of thiothixene with loxapine. J Clin Psychiatry. 1986;47(6):294–7.
54. Dubin WR, Waxman HM, Weiss KJ, Ramchandani D, Tavani-Petrone C. Rapid tranquilization: the efficacy of oral concentrate. J Clin Psychiatry. 1985;46(11):475–8.
55. NHS Camden & Islington NHS Trust. Rapid Tranquillisation Guidance (PHA03). London: National Healthcare System; 2019. https://www.candi.nhs.uk/sites/default/files/Rapid%20Tranquillisation%20Guidelines_PHA03_January%202019.pdf
56. Kleijer BC, van Marum RJ, Egberts AC, Jansen PA, Knol W, Heerdink ER. Risk of cerebrovascular events in elderly users of antipsychotics. J Psychopharmacol. 2009;23(8):909–14. https://doi.org/10.1177/0269881108093583.
57. Shin JY, Choi NK, Lee J, Seong JM, Park MJ, Lee SH, Park BJ. Risk of ischemic stroke associated with the use of antipsychotic drugs in elderly patients: a retrospective cohort study in Korea. PLoS One. 2015;10(3):e0119931. https://doi.org/10.1371/journal.pone.0119931.

58. Shaughnessy AF. Nonpharmacologic approaches are better than medication to control aggression and agitation in dementia. Am Fam Physician. 2020;101(10):631–2.
59. Kroll L, Böhning N, Müßigbrodt H, Stahl M, Halkin P, Liehr B, Grunow C, Kujumdshieva-Böhning B, Freise C, Hopfenmüller W, Friesdorf W, Jockers-Scherübl M, Somasundaram R. Non-contact monitoring of agitation and use of a sheltering device in patients with dementia in emergency departments: a feasibility study. BMC Psychiatry. 2020;20(1):165. https://doi.org/10.1186/s12888-020-02573-5.
60. Lozupone M, La Montagna M, Sardone R, Seripa D, Daniele A, Panza F. Can pharmacotherapy effectively reduce Alzheimer's related agitation? Expert Opin Pharmacother. 2020;21(13):1517–22. https://doi.org/10.1080/14656566.2020.1770730.
61. Stowell KR, Florence P, Harman HJ, Glick RL. Psychiatric evaluation of the agitated patient: consensus statement of the American Association for Emergency Psychiatry project Beta psychiatric evaluation workgroup. West J Emerg Med. 2012;13(1):11–6. https://doi.org/10.5811/westjem.2011.9.6868.
62. Huber CG, Lambert M, Naber D, Schacht A, Hundemer HP, Wagner TT, Schimmelmann BG. Validation of a Clinical Global Impression Scale for Aggression (CGI-A) in a sample of 558 psychiatric patients. Schizophr Res. 2008;100(1–3):342–8. https://doi.org/10.1016/j.schres.2007.12.480.
63. Hankin CS, Bronstone A, Koran LM. Agitation in the inpatient psychiatric setting: a review of clinical presentation, burden, and treatment. J Psychiatr Pract. 2011;17(3):170–85. https://doi.org/10.1097/01.pra.0000398410.21374.7d.
64. Bryan CJ, Hitschfeld MJ, Palmer BA, Schak KM, Roberge EM, Lineberry TW. Gender differences in the association of agitation and suicide attempts among psychiatric inpatients. Gen Hosp Psychiatry. 2014;36(6):726–31. https://doi.org/10.1016/j.genhosppsych.2014.09.013.
65. Eberhard J, Weiller E. Suicidality and symptoms of anxiety, irritability, and agitation in patients experiencing manic episodes with depressive symptoms: a naturalistic study. Neuropsychiatr Dis Treat. 2016;12:2265–71. https://doi.org/10.2147/NDT.S111094.
66. Fisher K, Houtsma C, Assavedo BL, Green BA, Anestis MD. Agitation as a moderator of the relationship between insomnia and current suicidal ideation in the military. Arch Suicide Res. 2017;21(4):531–43. https://doi.org/10.1080/13811118.2016.1193077.
67. McClure JR, Criqui MH, Macera CA, Ji M, Nievergelt CM, Zisook S. Prevalence of suicidal ideation and other suicide warning signs in veterans attending an urgent care psychiatric clinic. Compr Psychiatry. 2015;60:149–55. https://doi.org/10.1016/j.comppsych.2014.09.010.
68. Olgiati P, Serretti A, Colombo C. Retrospective analysis of psychomotor agitation, hypomanic symptoms, and suicidal ideation in unipolar depression. Depress Anxiety. 2006;23(7):389–97. https://doi.org/10.1002/da.20191.
69. Ribeiro JD, Bender TW, Selby EA, Hames JL, Joiner TE. Development and validation of a brief self-report measure of agitation: the brief agitation measure. J Pers Assess. 2011;93(6):597–604. https://doi.org/10.1080/00223891.2011.608758.
70. Sani G, Tondo L, Koukopoulos A, Reginaldi D, Kotzalidis GD, Koukopoulos AE, Manfredi G, Mazzarini L, Pacchiarotti I, Simonetti A, Ambrosi E, Angeletti G, Girardi P, Tatarelli R. Suicide in a large population of former psychiatric inpatients. Psychiatry Clin Neurosci. 2011;65(3):286–95. https://doi.org/10.1111/j.1440-1819.2011.02205.x.
71. Ferracuti S, Barchielli B, Napoli C, Fineschi V, Mandarelli G. Evaluation of official procedures for suicide prevention in hospital from a forensic psychiatric and a risk management perspective. Int J Psychiatry Clin Pract. 2020;24:24–245. https://doi.org/10.1080/13651501.2020.1759647.
72. Nordstrom K, Zun LS, Wilson MP, Stiebel V, Ng AT, Bregman B, Anderson EL. Medical evaluation and triage of the agitated patient: consensus statement of the American Association for Emergency Psychiatry project Beta medical evaluation workgroup. West J Emerg Med. 2012;13(1):3–10. https://doi.org/10.5811/westjem.2011.9.6863.
73. Allen MH, Currier GW, Hughes DH, Reyes-Harde M, Docherty JP. Expert consensus panel for behavioral emergencies. The expert consensus guideline series. Treatment of behavioral emergencies. Postgrad Med. 2001:1–88; quiz 89–90.

74. Yudofsky SC, Kopecky HJ, Kunik M, Silver JM, Endicott J. The Overt Agitation Severity Scale for the objective rating of agitation. J Neuropsychiatry Clin Neurosci. 1997;9(4):541–8. https://doi.org/10.1176/jnp.9.4.541.
75. DeBattista C, Solomon A, Arnow B, Kendrick E, Tilston J, Schatzberg AF. The efficacy of divalproex sodium in the treatment of agitation associated with major depression. J Clin Psychopharmacol. 2005;25(5):476–9. https://doi.org/10.1097/01.jcp.0000177552.21338.b0.
76. Jung S, Proske M, Kahl KG, Krüger TH, Wollmer MA. The new Hamburg-Hannover agitation scale in clinical samples: manifestation and differences of agitation in depression, anxiety, and borderline personality disorder. Psychopathology. 2016;49(6):420–8. https://doi.org/10.1159/000451029.
77. Kay SR, Fiszbein A, Opler LA. The positive and negative syndrome scale (PANSS) for schizophrenia. Schizophr Bull. 1987;13(2):261–76. https://doi.org/10.1093/schbul/13.2.261.
78. Battaglia J, Lindborg SR, Alaka K, Meehan K, Wright P. Calming versus sedative effects of intramuscular olanzapine in agitated patients. Am J Emerg Med. 2003;21:192–8. https://doi.org/10.1016/s0735-6757(02)42249-8.
79. De Filippis S, Cuomo I, Lionetto L, Janiri D, Simmaco M, Caloro M, De Persis S, Piazzi G, Simonetti A, Telesforo CL, Sciarretta A, Caccia F, Gentile G, Kotzalidis GD, Girardi P. Intramuscular aripiprazole in the acute management of psychomotor agitation. Pharmacotherapy. 2013;33(6):603–14. https://doi.org/10.1002/phar.1260.
80. Ostinelli EG, Jajawi S, Spyridi S, Sayal K, Jayaram MB. Aripiprazole (intramuscular) for psychosis-induced aggression or agitation (rapid tranquillisation). Cochrane Database Syst Rev. 2018;1(1):CD008074. https://doi.org/10.1002/14651858.CD008074.pub2.
81. Walther S, Moggi F, Horn H, Moskvitin K, Abderhalden C, Maier N, Strik W, Müller TJ. Rapid tranquilization of severely agitated patients with schizophrenia spectrum disorders: a naturalistic, rater-blinded, randomized, controlled study with oral haloperidol, risperidone, and olanzapine. J Clin Psychopharmacol. 2014;34(1):124–8. https://doi.org/10.1097/JCP.0000000000000050.
82. TREC Collaborative Group. Rapid tranquillisation for agitated patients in emergency psychiatric rooms: a randomised trial of midazolam versus haloperidol plus promethazine. BMJ. 2003;327(7417):708–13. https://doi.org/10.1136/bmj.327.7417.708.
83. Andrezina R, Marcus RN, Oren DA, Manos G, Stock E, Carson WH, McQuade RD. Intramuscular aripiprazole or haloperidol and transition to oral therapy in patients with agitation associated with schizophrenia: sub-analysis of a double-blind study. Curr Med Res Opin. 2006;22(11):2209–19. https://doi.org/10.1185/030079906X148445.
84. Huf G, Coutinho ES, Adams CE, TREC Collaborative Group. Rapid tranquillisation in psychiatric emergency settings in Brazil: pragmatic randomised controlled trial of intramuscular haloperidol versus intramuscular haloperidol plus promethazine. BMJ. 2007;335(7625):869. https://doi.org/10.1136/bmj.39339.448819.AE.
85. Wright P, Birkett M, David SR, Meehan K, Ferchland I, Alaka KJ, Saunders JC, Krueger J, Bradley P, San L, Bernardo M, Reinstein M, Breier A. Double-blind, placebo-controlled comparison of intramuscular olanzapine and intramuscular haloperidol in the treatment of acute agitation in schizophrenia. Am J Psychiatry. 2001;158(7):1149–51. https://doi.org/10.1176/appi.ajp.158.7.1149.
86. Richards JR, Derlet RW, Duncan DR. Chemical restraint for the agitated patient in the emergency department: lorazepam versus droperidol. J Emerg Med. 1998;16(4):567–73. https://doi.org/10.1016/s0736-4679(98)00045-6.
87. Taylor DMD, Yap CYL, Knott JC, Taylor SE, Phillips GA, Karro J, Chan EW, Kong DCM, Castle DJ. Midazolam-droperidol, droperidol, or olanzapine for acute agitation: a randomized clinical trial. Ann Emerg Med. 2017;69(3):318–326.e1. https://doi.org/10.1016/j.annemergmed.2016.07.033.
88. Cester-Martínez A, Cortés-Ramas JA, Borraz-Clares D, Pellicer-Gayarre M. Inhaled loxapine for the treatment of psychiatric agitation in the prehospital setting: a case series. Clin Pract Cases Emerg Med. 2017;1(4):345–8. https://doi.org/10.5811/cpcem.2017.5.33840.

89. Patel MX, Sethi FN, Barnes TR, Dix R, Dratcu L, Fox B, Garriga M, Haste JC, Kahl KG, Lingford-Hughes A, McAllister-Williams H, O'Brien A, Parker C, Paterson B, Paton C, Posporelis S, Taylor DM, Vieta E, Völlm B, Wilson-Jones C, Woods L. Joint BAP NAPICU evidence-based consensus guidelines for the clinical management of acute disturbance: de-escalation and rapid tranquillisation. J Psychopharmacol. 2018;32(6):601–40. https://doi.org/10.1177/0269881118776738.
90. Calver L, Drinkwater V, Isbister GK. A prospective study of high dose sedation for rapid tranquilisation of acute behavioural disturbance in an acute mental health unit. BMC Psychiatry. 2013;13:225. https://doi.org/10.1186/1471-244X-13-225.
91. Mantovani C, Labate CM, Sponholz A Jr, de Azevedo Marques JM, Guapo VG, de Simone Brito dos Santos ME, Pazin-Filho A, Del-Ben CM. Are low doses of antipsychotics effective in the management of psychomotor agitation? A randomized, rated-blind trial of 4 intramuscular interventions. J Clin Psychopharmacol. 2013;33(3):306–12. https://doi.org/10.1097/JCP.0b013e3182900fd6.
92. Zimbroff DL, Marcus RN, Manos G, Stock E, McQuade RD, Auby P, Oren DA. Management of acute agitation in patients with bipolar disorder: efficacy and safety of intramuscular aripiprazole. J Clin Psychopharmacol. 2007;27(2):171–6. https://doi.org/10.1097/JCP.0b13e318033bd5e.
93. Tran-Johnson TK, Sack DA, Marcus RN, Auby P, McQuade RD, Oren DA. Efficacy and safety of intramuscular aripiprazole in patients with acute agitation: a randomized, double-blind, placebo-controlled trial. J Clin Psychiatry. 2007;68(1):111–9. https://doi.org/10.4088/jcp.v68n0115.
94. Horsfall JT, Sprague JE. The pharmacology and toxicology of the 'Holy Trinity'. Basic Clin Pharmacol Toxicol. 2017;120(2):115–9. https://doi.org/10.1111/bcpt.12655.
95. American Psychiatric Association. Diagnostic and statistical manual of mental disorders, third edition-revised (DSM-III-R). Washington, DC: American Psychiatric Publishing; 1987.
96. Gutheil TG. Restraint versus treatment: seclusion as discussed in the Boston State Hospital case. Am J Psychiatry. 1980;137(6):718–9. https://doi.org/10.1176/ajp.137.6.718.
97. Tasić M, Simić M, Radić A, Zivojnović S, Vujić D. Fatal central effects of diazepam potentiated by alcohol and haldol. Acta Med Leg Soc (Liège). 1985;35(1):185–9.
98. Khokhar MA, Rathbone J. Droperidol for psychosis-induced aggression or agitation. Cochrane Database Syst Rev. 2016;12(12):CD002830. https://doi.org/10.1002/14651858.CD002830.pub3.
99. Huang CL, Hwang TJ, Chen YH, Huang GH, Hsieh MH, Chen HH, Hwu HG. Intramuscular olanzapine versus intramuscular haloperidol plus lorazepam for the treatment of acute schizophrenia with agitation: an open-label, randomized controlled trial. J Formos Med Assoc. 2015;114(5):438–45. https://doi.org/10.1016/j.jfma.2015.01.018.

Communication in Psychiatric Coercive Treatment and Patients' Decisional Capacity to Consent

Gabriele Mandarelli and Giovanna Parmigiani

7.1 Introduction

A good doctor-patient relationship relies on several components such as verbal and nonverbal communication, expression of empathy and concern, and sufficient transmission of information to allow the patient's active participation in the decisional process during the informed consent acquisition [1]. Effective communication is central in patient's comprehension of treatment benefits and risks and increases compliance [2].

Among the factors contributing to hindering doctor-patient communication, the doctor's fear to become excessively involved in the relationship and worries about not being able to solve and manage the patient's emotions or to unnecessarily hurt the patient have been mentioned. This issue becomes even more tricky, when it comes to breaking bad news, a task which has been shown to have an impact both on the deliver and the recipient [3].

In recent years, several efforts have been done to improve communication skills of health professionals, such as the six-step SPIKES, the ABCED, and the BROKE strategy, designed for breaking bad news [4]. Among these, one of the most acknowledged is the model developed by Buckman [5] that explains every step that the clinician must follow when communicating a diagnosis and is referred to with the acronym of SPIKES (see Fig. 7.1). The author sustained that the effect of the bad news depends on the difference between the patient's

G. Mandarelli (✉)
Interdisciplinary Department of Medicine, University of Bari "Aldo Moro", Bari, Italy
e-mail: gabriele.mandarelli@uniba.it

G. Parmigiani
Department of Neurosciences, Mental Health and Sensory Organs,
University of Rome "Sapienza", Rome, Italy
e-mail: giovanna.parmigiani@uniroma1.it

© Springer Nature Switzerland AG 2021
M. Biondi et al. (eds.), *Empathy, Normalization and De-escalation*,
https://doi.org/10.1007/978-3-030-65106-0_7

Step 1: S—Setting up the interview
- Arrange for some privacy
- Involve significant others
- Sit down
- Make connection and establish rapport with the patient
- Manage time constraints and interruptions

Step 2: P—Assessing the patient's perception of condition/seriousness
- Determine what the patient knows about the medical condition or what he suspects.
- Listen to the patient's level of comprehension
- Accept denial but do not confront at this stage

Step 3: I—Invitation from the patient to give information
- Ask patient if s/he wishes to know the details of the medical condition and/or treatment
- Accept patient's right not to know
- Offer to answer questions later if s/he wishes

Step 4: K—Giving knowledge and information to the patient
- Use language intelligible to patient
- Consider educational level, socio-cultural background, current emotional state
- Give information in small chunks
- Check whether the patient understood what you said
- Respond to the patient's reactions as they occur
- Give any positive aspects first e.g.: Cancer has not spread to lymph nodes, highly responsive to therapy, treatment available locally, etc.
- Give facts accurately about treatment options, prognosis, costs etc.

Step 5: E—Addressing the patient's emotions with empathic responses
- Prepare to give an empathetic response:
  1. Identify emotion expressed by the patient (sadness, silence, shock, etc.)
  2. Identify cause/ source of emotion
  3. Give the patient time to express his or her feelings, and then respond in a way that demonstrates you have recognized connection between 1 and 2.

Step 6: S—Strategy and summary
- Close the interview
- Ask whether they want to clarify something else
- Offer agenda for the next meeting eg: I will speak to you again when we have the opinion of cancer specialist

Fig. 7.1 SPIKES: a six-step strategy for breaking bad news [6]

expectations and the reality of the situation. However, the common belief that receiving unfavourable medical information invariably causes psychological harm is unfounded. Most patients expect truthful medical information to help them making decisions that are relevant for their lives [6]. In North America principles of informed consent, patient's autonomy and case law have established ethical and legal obligations to provide patients with as much information as they desire about their illness and its treatment [7].

7.2   Patients' Decisional Capacity to Consent to Medical Treatment

Valid informed consent requires the satisfaction of three main criteria: full information; voluntary participation; and patients' capacity to make a decision [8]. Capacity to consent to treatment is a multidimensional construct and relies on several abilities [9, 10], such as understanding and appreciating information, reasoning, and expressing a choice [8] (see Fig. 7.2). Several tools have been developed to assist clinicians when evaluating patients' capacity to consent to treatment, among which the most widely used is the *MacArthur Competence Assessment Tool for Treatment* (MacCAT-T) [11].

Among vulnerable populations at risk of impaired capacity to consent to treatment are psychiatric patients. Psychotic disorders, particularly schizophrenia, are associated with reduced ability to adequately decide about treatment [11–15], although a considerable variability in individual capacity has been reported [9, 13, 14, 16–18]. Hence, a diagnosis of a mental disorder is not a label of incapacity. Psychiatric inpatients do not necessarily perform poorer than medical inpatients in informed consent decision-making measures [19], and significant within-group variability has emerged in both groups of patients [20–22].

A risk of impaired capacity to consent to treatment has often been associated with specific clinical characteristics [23]; among these are excitement and positive symptoms [24–27] together with the severity of psychiatric symptoms [25],

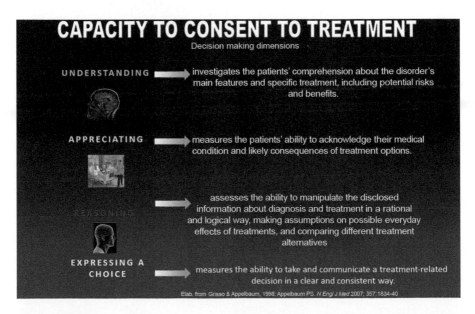

Fig. 7.2 Capacity to consent to treatment. (Elaboration from Grisso & Appelbaum, 1998; Appelbaum, 2007)

cognitive dysfunction [9, 13, 28], especially impaired executive functioning [29]. In addition, multiple environmental factors may play a role in determining the variability of patients' capacity to consent to treatment or research participation [18, 30], including the complexity of disclosed information, type of clinical setting, and quality of consent forms and disclosing procedures (see Fig. 7.3).

Patients affected by schizophrenia and bipolar disorder show a wide array of specific cognitive and neuropsychological alterations in working memory, verbal memory, information processing speed, attention, sensory processing, and executive functioning that have been described since the early stages of the disorders [31–33]. Multiple domains of mental functioning, most of which appear to rely on the concept of executive functions, such as will, inhibition, abstract reasoning, concept formation, prediction, and planning, are involved in the decisional process [34].

Executive functions rely upon frontal-cortical areas together with other complex networks of frontal-cortical and subcortical circuitries and play a role in cognitive set shifts and in learning new rules in accordance with varying environmental feedbacks, accounting altogether for the cognitive flexibility of the individual [35]. Because all these features are encompassed by complex decision-making processes, such as those involved in informed consent acquisition, executive functions may intuitively be involved in this context, and executive dysfunction might play a significant role in determining incompetency.

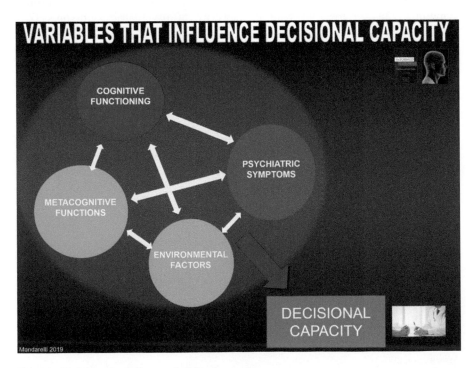

Fig. 7.3 Variables that influence decisional capacity

An association between executive functions and consent process has already been reported by four studies [10, 29, 36, 37], while one did not [34]. Differences in methods and study samples may account for the lack of clear evidence. For instance, Koren and colleagues [34] did not observe any correlation between executive functions investigated by the Wisconsin Card Sorting Test (WCST) and patients' competence to consent to treatment; however, they did observe a role for metacognition. Conversely another study [36] found that incompetent patients scored significantly poorer than competent ones at the executive interview [38].

In a study [29] aimed at investigating the association between executive functions and capacity to consent to treatment, we enrolled a sample of psychiatric inpatients hospitalized in the Psychiatric Intensive Care Unit of the Hospital Policlinico Umberto I of Rome. Patients with poor executive functions, measured through the WCST performed worse in MacCAT-T understanding, appreciation, and expression of a choice, compared with those with good WCST scores, a result which underlined the role of executive functions in decisional capacity processes. The significant associations between learning abilities and informed consent decision-making provided empirical evidence indicating possible cognitive enhancement strategies that may improve psychiatric patients' competency.

7.3   Informed Consent in Involuntary Psychiatric Treatment

Despite the differences in the legal framework for involuntary hospitalization in different countries, the abilities required for giving a valid informed consent/dissent to treatment are well recognized [8].

A systematic review by Okai and colleagues [39] reported that involuntary psychiatric patients were at a higher risk of incapacity compared to their voluntary counterparts. However, the few studies which have been performed on involuntary hospitalized patients' decisional capacity led to discrepant results, probably due to methodological problems including heterogeneous study samples and assessment methods [40–43]. Some authors reported no significant differences in treatment decision-making capacity between psychiatric patients admitted voluntarily or involuntarily [43], while others found that an involuntarily admitted subgroup scored worse on a scale measuring information understanding [44]. Yet others reported that a small sample of patients detained under the Mental Health Act 1983 lacked mental capacity to decide about hospital admission [40] and treatment [41].

A study on a mixed sample of voluntary and detained inpatients using the MacCAT-T found that 43.8% of all inpatients lacked capacity and 9.5% of detained patients had competence to consent to treatment [26]. The presence of mania, psychosis, delusions, and poor insight was among the clinical factors associated with incapacity [26]. In more recent years, Owen and colleagues found that 60% (95% CI 55–65) among 338 patients hospitalized in 3 general adult acute psychiatric inpatient units lacked mental capacity to make treatment decisions [27], with patients with mania or being detained having higher rates of incapacity.

In a study [24] on a sample of acute psychiatric patients hospitalized at the University Hospital Policlinico Umberto I of Rome, we found significant differences in capacity to consent to treatment between involuntarily and voluntarily hospitalized patients. Involuntarily treated patients as a group performed significantly worse than their voluntary counterparts in all MacCAT-T measures. They appeared less able to understand and appreciate their own clinical condition, the risks, and benefits of treatment and less able to reason about it, or express a clear treatment choice, compared to their voluntarily counterpart.

Despite the poorer MacCAT-T performances identified in involuntarily patients, both study groups showed great variability, particularly in MacCAT-T *understanding* and *appreciation* scores. Unexpectedly, up to 30% of patients treated involuntarily understood the disclosed information about treatment well or extremely well. Most surprisingly, the same percentage of involuntary patients scored 3 or 4 at appreciation, thus indicating that they completely or almost completely acknowledged their medical condition as well as the consequences of possible treatment options. However, their reasoning abilities were severely impaired. More than half of the patients admitted involuntarily were judged incapable of rationally arguing about how psychiatric treatment or possibly no treatment affected their everyday life (see Fig. 7.4). This unexpected intragroup variability probably depends on the multidimensional framework we used for evaluating capacity to consent to treatment [8, 39, 45]. Our data seem to suggest that lack of treatment-related decisional capacity is a common but by no means inevitable correlate of admission to a psychiatric inpatient unit [26, 27]. Accordingly, in our study, some involuntary patients understood all the essential information they received about treatment, yet they were treated involuntarily. We attribute their impaired capacity mainly to altered reasoning abilities. Conversely, within the voluntary study sample, up to 27% patients agreed neither with their diagnosis, nor with the type of treatment they were receiving, as indicated by a score of 0 at *appreciation*, a feature usually found in people incapable of giving valid informed consent. These findings support Owen

Fig. 7.4 Capacity to consent to treatment in involuntarily and voluntarily hospitalized patients

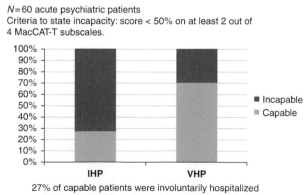

$N = 60$ acute psychiatric patients
Criteria to state incapacity: score < 50% on at least 2 out of 4 MacCAT-T subscales.

27% of capable patients were involuntarily hospitalized
30 % of incapable patients were volutarily treated

IHP = involuntarily hospitalized patients
VHP = voluntarily hospitalized patients

et al.'s [27] suggestion that mental capacity or incapacity to make treatment decisions cannot be presumed and may not overlap with capacity as measured by validated capacity assessments.

Involuntary treatment was associated with more manic symptoms, as disclosed by conditional stepwise logistic regression analysis. The role of psychiatric symptoms in determining incapacity in an acute psychiatric setting has been already underlined in non-forensic [25–27] and forensic psychiatric samples [46]. In interpreting this result, we must consider that involuntary psychiatric treatment was decided before study recruitment, relying on a non-capacity-based law. In the regression analysis, we found no association between cognitive measures and voluntariness of hospitalization and treatment. A possible explanation of this result relies in the possible prominent effect of severe psychiatric symptoms in acute psychiatric inpatients, such as those we studied, which might largely override the possible effect of cognition in determining capacity levels. We selected involuntary patients according to the Italian civil jurisdiction since we wanted specifically to focus on those patients who needed treatment for an acute mental disorder in a real-world clinical setting.

In a second phase, we performed a multicentre study on 131 acute non-forensic involuntary treated patients to investigate acute non-consensual psychiatric patients' treatment decision-making capacities (DMC) in a representative sample from three distinct Italian regions [47]. We classified patients as having high or low treatment DMC and found a significant variability in their degree of impairment in treatment DMC. Decisional impairment was a common but not always unavoidable characteristic of patients involuntary hospitalized in the acute psychiatric inpatient units, which is in line with previous initial research on smaller samples from single centres [24, 26, 27].

Twenty-two percent of the 131 patients scored >75% on every MacCAT-T subscale and were classified as having high treatment DMC. Patients affected by schizophrenia and schizophreniform disorder performed worst on DMC. The percentage of patients with high treatment DMC reached 32% among bipolar disorder patients and 42% among other diagnoses, such as personality disorders. Regarding the latter group, they showed an almost complete understanding and appreciating of their clinical condition, as well as of the risks and benefits of their treatment (or no treatment), an adequate capacity to reason about their therapy and to express a choice (i.e. no hospitalization/treatment) in a clear and consistent way.

The result was surprising and has implications for researchers, clinical psychiatrists, and policymakers as it seems to imply that under the Italian mental health regulation, or a need for care regulation, a capable patients' refusal of treatment can be overridden for reasons that are not of immediate understanding and deserves further consideration. A possible explanation would be the implicit application of a "best interest" criterion in which capable patients' refusal was overridden in their interest. Nonetheless this would contrast with the principle of autonomy. Another possible explanation is that physician decision-making included a *dangerousness* criterion, even though the Italian law does not require it, for example, in case of actual suicide risk. Finally, we should consider that patients' treatment DMC could vary fast in acute psychiatric settings. Even though we assessed patients within 3 days from admission, it could be possible that treatment DMC had significantly improved due to hospitalization and to pharmacological treatment. Therefore, the patients' DMC level assessed during this study could have been different from the one displayed when physicians decided involuntary admission. This hypothesis deserves future studies aimed at investigating rapid changes in treatment DMC in acute inpatients since it would have implications also under a capacity-based mental health legislation.

The finding of a poorer treatment DMC in patients affected by schizophrenia spectrum disorder compared to patients affected by bipolar disorder questions existing data indicating a minor role for diagnoses rather than symptoms. For example, Palmer and colleagues [48] found no differences between long-term illness outpatients affected by bipolar disorder and long-term illness outpatients affected by schizophrenia in competence to consent to research, as measured through the MacCAT-CR. Howe and colleagues [25] found no differences in MacCAT-T scores between acute psychiatric patients affected by schizophrenia, schizoaffective, and bipolar disorder (manic/mixed phase). However, the result we report here suggests that schizophrenia spectrum disorder patients are at greater risk of impaired treatment DMC in acute coercive psychiatric settings.

Greater impairment of treatment DMC was associated with the severity of positive symptoms in the sample overall, acute mania in bipolar disorder patients, and cognitive impairment in schizophrenia spectrum disorder patients.

7.4 Doctor-Patient Communication in Coercive Medical Settings

Coercive practices, ranging from subtle to overt coercion, are quite common in psychiatry. Among these are included involuntary admission, forced pharmacological treatments, and physical restraint, which are usually referred to as *objective coercion*, to be distinguished from *perceived coercion*, described as the subjective experience of being coerced when receiving treatment. In the mental health setting, feeling coerced has been described as perceiving that one does not have influence, control, freedom, or choice or does not make the decision to enter the hospital [49], and it has been reported also from those patients who have not been subjected to objective coercive measures [50–52].

As is the case of objective coercion, the subjective experience of being coerced may have several clinical implications. A poorer prognosis, a higher number of relapses and rehospitalization, as well as lower adherence to treatment has been linked to higher perceived coercion [53, 54]. The subjective experience of being forced significantly decreases with the improvement in global functioning and the reduction of positive symptoms [55, 56] and seems to not predict engagement with follow-up [50, 57]. Nonetheless, other studies showed no clear association between clinical variables such as symptoms of psychoticism or depression and clear signs of hostility and perceived coercion [58, 59].

Efforts to define the concrete implementation and lessening of coercive intervention in clinical practice have been made [60, 61]. The MacArthur Research Network on Mental Health and the Law [62] has developed an instrument, the Admission Experience Survey (AES), designed to assess psychiatric patients' perception of their hospitalization experience, including their perceived coercion. The AES is composed of 15 items, in a true-false format. It contains three subscales covering (a) "perceived coercion" (composed of items focusing on influence, control, choice, freedom, and idea, ranging from 0 to 5, where a score of 5 reflects the maximum degree of subjective coercion); (b) "perceived negative pressures" (composed of six items, evaluating if in the process of hospitalization threats and force were applied, ranging from 0 to 6); and (c) "voice" (composed of four items assessing to what extent patients experienced that they had a chance to speak—voice—and having others take into account their viewpoints—validation).

The AES has been used in different countries [50–52, 55–57, 62–66] and proved useful for measuring subjective coercion in different psychiatric clinical settings [62]. We performed the Italian translation and validation of the AES [1] (see Fig. 7.5) on a sample of 156 acutely admitted psychiatric patients, the 31.4% ($n = 49$) of whom were involuntarily committed. The factorial analysis of the I-AES disclosed a three-factor solution (Table 7.1) explaining 59.3 of the total variance. The three factors were as follows:

1. Perceived coercion
2. External pressure
3. Choice expression

The I-AES showed good internal consistency (Cronbach's alpha = 0.90); Guttmann split-half reliability coefficient was 0.90.

In line with previous studies [50, 51, 67], in our sample involuntarily committed patients tended to feel more coerced during admission compared to voluntarily committed ones, despite perceived coercion being present in both groups. In both groups of patients, perceived coercion was associated with the number of previous involuntary commitments. This may be interpreted bearing in mind that patients with a history of a higher number of previous involuntary hospitalizations tend to have more severe psychiatric symptoms and to be less compliant with treatment and more aversive towards psychiatric care, thus probably resulting in the experience of feeling more coerced during hospital admission.

The severity of psychiatric symptoms was positively correlated with perceived coercion. Specifically, the presence of manic symptoms was associated with a higher subjective coercion, with patients reporting more threats and force application during the process of hospitalization together with a lower chance to have a say in the admission or having others take into account their viewpoints. This is not surprising, bearing in mind that often in psychiatric practice patients affected by bipolar disorder in a manic phase tend to totally lack insight and are often admitted on an involuntary basis. In other studies, the presence of mania was associated with both the involuntary commitment status and a poorer capacity to consent to

(Versione originale di: Gardner W. *et al.* Behavioral Sciences and the Law. 1993;20:307-321, traduzione di Gabriele Mandarelli)

Identificativo paziente:....................................Data valutazione: ..../............./.........................

"Sto per leggerle alcune affermazioni riguardo il suo attuale ricovero in ospedale. Le chiedo di rispondere "vero" o "falso" per ogni affermazione. Cerchi di rispondere individualmente ad ogni singola domanda, non importa quantole possa sembrare simile alle altre."

	VERO	FALSO	NON SO
1. Mi sono sentito libero di fare ciò che volevo circa il venire in ospedale	☐	☐	☐
2. Alcune persone hanno provato a forzarmi a venire in ospedale	☐	☐	☐
3. Ho avuto sufficienti possibilità di dire se volevo venire in ospedale o no	☐	☐	☐
4. Ho scelto io di venire in ospedale	☐	☐	☐
5. Sono riuscito a dire quello che volevo, a proposito del venire in ospedale	☐	☐	☐
6. Qualcuno mi ha minacciato per farmi venire in ospedale	☐	☐	☐
7. Venire in ospedale è stata una mia idea	☐	☐	☐
8. Qualcuno ha cercato di forzarmi fisicamente a venire in ospedale	☐	☐	☐
9. Nessuno è sembrato interessato a sapere se io volessi venire in ospedale, oppure no	☐	☐	☐
10. Hanno minacciato di ricoverarmi	☐	☐	☐
11. Mi hanno detto che mi avrebbero fatto venire in ospedale	☐	☐	☐
12. Nessuno ha provato a forzarmi a venire in ospedale	☐	☐	☐
13. La mia opinione circa il venire in ospedale non ha contato nulla	☐	☐	☐
14. Ho avuto molto controllo sulla decisione di andare in ospedale	☐	☐	☐
15. Sono stato io a decidere, più di chiunque altro, se venirein ospedale o no	☐	☐	☐
16. Come la ha fatta sentire essere ricoverato/a in ospedale?			
a) Arrabbiato/a	☐	☐	☐
b) Triste	☐	☐	☐
c) Soddisfatto/a	☐	☐	☐
d) Sollevato/a			
e) Confuso/a	☐	☐	☐
f) Impaurito/a	☐	☐	☐
	☐	☐	☐

Fig. 7.5 Admission Experience Survey, Italian version (I-AES)

Table 7.1 I-AES principal component analysis

Admission experience survey items	Perceived coercion (Factor 1)	External pressure (Factor 2)	Choice expression (Factor 3)
7. It was my idea to come into the hospital	0.78		
15. I had more influence than anyone else on whether I came into the hospital	0.73		
4. I chose to come into the hospital	0.69		
1. I felt free to do what I wanted about coming into the hospital	0.63		
13. My opinion about coming into the hospital didn't matter	0.60		
14. I had a lot of control over whether I went into the hospital	0.59		
2. People tried to force me to come into the hospital		0.51	
11. They said they would make me come into the hospital	0.50		
10. I was threatened with commitment		0.86	
6. Someone threatened me to get me to come into the hospital		0.79	
8. Someone physically tried to make me come into the hospital		0.63	
12. No one tried to force me to come into the hospital		0.53	
5. I got to say what I wanted about coming into the hospital			0.75
3. I had enough of a chance to say whether I wanted to come into the hospital			0.67
9. No one seemed to want to know whether I wanted to come into the hospital			0.60
Cronbach's alpha	0.84	0.79	0.71
Variance explained	25.1	19.1	15.1

treatment [24, 47]. It would be interesting to investigate the presence of an association between perceived coercion and capacity to consent to treatment in clinical populations and how cognitive and psychiatric symptoms play a role in this picture. Anxiety and depressive symptoms were negatively associated with perceived coercion and external/negative pressure, probably because patients affected by depression are more inclined to voluntarily or passively adhere to psychiatric treatment and hospital admission. Finally, negative symptoms were associated with a higher perception of coercion, while positive symptoms were associated with the experience of external/negative pressure. This last result may be explained by the fact that probably patients with a distorted perception of their disease tend to consider hospitalization as an inadequate measure, consequently feeling more coerced in the clinical setting.

7.5   Involuntary Psychiatric Hospitalization

Despite the significant efforts towards reducing the coercion associated with treatment of severe mental disorders, coercive measures, such as involuntary psychiatric hospitalization (IPH), are often regarded as an inevitable and yet highly debated feature of psychiatric care. Several concerns have been raised about the implications of non-consensual psychiatric care in terms of possible violations of personal rights, as well as limitations of personal autonomy [63, 64].

In Italy, IPH is regulated by Law 833 of 1978, which assimilated the so-called Basaglia Law, as part of the deinstitutionalization process of civil psychiatric care. Under the Law 833, civil mental hospitals were replaced by a range of community-based psychiatric services and by psychiatric wards in general hospitals for acute inpatient care [68], with no more than 15 beds each, to prevent the establishment of large-scale, asylum-like wards [69, 70]. The transition from a dangerousness criterion for involuntary civil hospitalization to a need for treatment one was also established. Specifically, three conditions are required for IPH in Italy: (1) the patient is suffering from psychic alterations that need immediate treatment; (2) the patient refuses that treatment; and (3) the patient cannot be adequately treated by other non-hospital-based means. Two medical doctors, not necessarily psychiatrists, must perform patients' evaluation and provide a proposal and a confirmation certificate, respectively. The second physician, who should verify and confirm the presence of all the criteria, must be an employee of the National Health Service. The IPH ordinance is issued by the city mayor, within 48 h following the confirmation certificate. The IPH ordinance is then further verified by the tutelary judge, which exercises a form of legal guarantee, within the 48 h following IPH. Maximum length of initial placement is 7 days, but it can be repeatedly extended for further 7 days upon a motivated medical decision certifying the persistence of the three abovementioned criteria.

This procedure allows compulsory placement and treatment. The evaluation of the capacity to make informed decisions is not a prerequisite, despite some studies having underlined that a percentage of involuntarily hospitalized psychiatric patients retains their mental capacity to consent to treatment [24, 47]. In addition, the law requires that from the beginning of involuntary admission, the doctors should pursue initiatives aimed at ensuring patient's consent and participation to the treatment choices. Anyone can appeal against the IPH decision. Private facilities are not allowed to perform IPH.

International data from a study comparing annual incidence of IPH between 2008 and 2017 in 22 countries across Europe, Australia, and New Zealand found that the median rate of IPH was 106.4 (IQR 58.5–150.9) per 100,000 individuals, with Austria having the highest (282 per 100,000), while Italy showed the lowest rates (14.5 per 100,000) [71]. A lower rate of absolute poverty, higher gross domestic product per capita, healthcare spending per capita, a higher proportion of foreign-born individuals in a population, and a large number of inpatient beds has been associated with a higher incidence of IPH [71]. No evidence linking rates of IPH to differences in legislation was found [71, 72].

Mental illness and danger-criterion	Austria, Belgium, France, Germany, Luxembourg, The Netherlands
Mental illness and danger-criterion *or* Mental illness and need for treatment-criterion	Denmark, Finland, Greece, Ireland, United kingdom, Portugal
Mental illness and need for treatment-criterion	Italy, Spain, Sweden

Fig. 7.6 Criteria for involuntary hospitalization in European countries (from Dressing & Salize, 2004)

In European countries, there are three main criteria for IPH: (a) mental illness and danger criterion (Austria, Belgium, France, Germany, Luxemburg, and the Netherlands); (b) mental illness and danger or need for treatment criterion (Denmark, Finland, Greece, Ireland, the UK Portugal); and (c) mental illness and need for treatment criterion (Italy, Spain, and Sweden) [73] (see Fig. 7.6).

Despite the wide variation in IPH rates across countries [72, 74], the clinical and socio-demographic characteristics of IPH patients are similar. Specifically, IPH is commonly associated with a diagnosis of psychosis [75–77], severity of psychiatric symptoms [78], male gender [79], low socioeconomic status [80], and reduced insight [81]. In Italy, the PROGRES-Acute project [82] showed that more than one-half of involuntary hospitalizations involved patients affected by schizophrenia spectrum disorders, whereas approximately one-fifth of the IPH patients was affected by bipolar disorder and one-tenth by personality disorder. Depressive or anxiety disorders accounted for a very small percentage among IPH patients [82].

We analysed 2796 case files between January 2013 and May 2016 deposited at the Office of the Tutelary Judge of the Civil Court of Rome, within a catchment area of 2,863,322 residents [83]. The IPH prevalence in the city of Rome was relatively low, showing a reduction over the years examined: from 3.04 per 10,000 people in 2013 to 2.60 per 10,000 people in 2015. A study by Gaddini and colleagues [84] conducted in the city of Rome in 2002 showed an approximate admission rate to acute psychiatric wards, including voluntarily and involuntarily admitted patients, of 31.8 per 10,000 residents. The low Italian rate of IPH has been underlined by another study [71], suggesting that this result might be due to the reduction in bed capacity established by the Law 180, as well as the presence of a culture which values deinstitutionalization and reintegration in the community.

For every 100,000 inhabitants, Italy has 46 psychiatric beds, as compared with 58 in the UK and 77 in the USA [68]. In interpreting these results, it is also possible to consider that an efficient psychiatric community care could account for a lower IPH rate.

There is evidence that most of the IPH proposal certificates in Italy include symptoms or diagnoses referring to schizophrenia spectrum disorders, which is a result confirmed by other studies on IPH [24, 47, 75, 77, 82]. A significantly higher frequency of violent or aggressive behaviour was found in IPH male patients compared to their female counterparts, who tended to present higher percentage of bipolar spectrum disorders or manic symptoms. An association between involuntary admission, male gender, and aggressiveness has been also underlined [85], such as the role of excitement symptoms in predicting compulsory admission [86].

Our results, based on the analysis of 2796 case files, showed that administrative issues are among the main reasons that prevent the tutelary judge from validating the IPH, an event which occurred only in the 0.8% of cases. Although our country provides for guaranteed measures to avoid improper restrictions of personal freedom and autonomy, as well as to ensure the protection of the rights of patients affected by mental disorders, these seem to only partially fulfil the proposed tasks. This may be due to the limited possibility of the magistrate to enter into the merits of eminently clinical decisions. In addition, up to 2.2% of the certificates were motivated on the only bases of the dangerousness criterion, occurrence that, in a legal system that explicitly requires the need of treatment, prompts a reflection and suggests a revision of the legal criteria currently applied in our country.

7.6   Improving Medical Communication

A good doctor-patient communication and the acquisition of valid informed consent are central to the doctor-patient relationship and a clinician's ethical obligation in order to respect patients' autonomy, as well as their right to be involved in treatment decisions [87]. In order to achieve valid informed consent acquisition, the information provided must be complete and adapted to the patient's sociocultural background, the participation must be voluntary, and the patient must be capable to make a decision.

Apart from psychiatric disorders, there are many diseases that can place patients at risk for impaired decisional capacity [88]. Some strategies have been suggested to maximize patients' capacities, such as (a) performing the evaluation in the patient's native language; (b) identifying and correcting potentially treatable conditions, such as fever, sedation, dehydration, depression, and anxiety, that may impair capacity; (c) manipulating the environment—for example, assessing patients affected by mild dementia early in the day to avoid sundowning or conducting consent discussions in quiet areas free from distractions; and (d) enhancing the informed consent process to make the decisional task easier [89]. In the last years, several efforts have been made in order to develop educational interventions to enhance psychiatric and non-psychiatric patients' decisional capacity [88]. A recent meta-analysis by Hostiuc and colleagues [90] found that enhanced informed consent forms can decrease decisional capacity differences between patients affected or not by psychaitric disorders.

Wang and colleagues [91], after developing and administering a 1-week informed consent information training process for improving competence to provide consent in stable community patients with schizophrenia, found that patients' decisional capacity could be improved after 1 week of training. Nonetheless such improvement was no longer observed 1 year later. Moser and colleagues [92], after the administration of a brief educational intervention to a sample of patients affected by schizophrenia, found that their performance was no longer significantly different from the healthy comparison group on any of the four dimensions of decisional capacity. Palmer and colleagues [93], in a study employing multimedia disclosure and cognitive feedback to improve decisional capacity among patients affected by Alzheimer disease (AD) and non-psychiatric comparison participants, found no significant effect of the enhanced consent procedure compared to routine consent. Another study by Mittal and colleagues [94], providing two enhanced consent procedures—a PowerPoint presentation and an enhanced printed consent form—to patients with AD or mild cognitive impairment, found an improvement in understanding in both conditions. However, this study yielded equivocal results due to the small sample size and the absence of a routine consent comparison condition. Finally, Rubright and colleagues [95] observed that a memory and organizational aid added to a standard consent procedure improved capacity to consent to research in patients affected by AD.

7.7   Conclusion

Based on our professional and research experience, a good doctor-patient communication and valid informed consent acquisition are often hindered by several issues among which the clinician's fear of hurting the patient by communicating a bad diagnosis or not knowing how to manage the patient's emotional reactions. Consequently, clinicians often disclose half-truths to the patient, or might limit themselves to informing family members about the real situation, instead of directly communicating with the patient.

The tools currently available to assess patients' decisional capacity during informed consent acquisition, which are mainly used in research contexts, could provide a helpful framework to be used on a routine basis when communicating diagnosis and treatment to the patients. The multidimensional decisional capacity model, as well as the semi-structured interview approach of the MacCAT-T, helps bringing the clinician and the patient together in a process of shared decision-making. Such approach can lead the patient to become actively involved in his/her treatment decisions. The presence of severe mental disorders proved not to be obstructing to a shared decision-making therapeutic process, even though the risk of patients' incapacity should be carefully accounted.

References

1. Roter DL, Frankel RM, Hall JA, Sluyter D. The expression of emotion through nonverbal behavior in medical visits. Mechanisms and outcomes. J Gen Intern Med. 2006;21(Suppl 1):S28–34.
2. Zolnierek KBH, Dimatteo MR. Physician communication and patient adherence to treatment: a meta-analysis. Med Care. 2009;47(8):826–34.
3. Amiel GE, Ungar L, Alperin M, Baharier Z, Cohen R, Reis S. Ability of primary care physicians to break bad news: a performance based assessment of an educational intervention. Patient Educ Couns. 2006;60:10–5.
4. Girgis A, Sanson-Fisher RW. Breaking bad news: consensus guidelines for medical practitioners. J Clin Oncol. 1995;13:2449–56.

5. Buckman R, Yvonne K. How to break bad news: a guide for health care professionals. Toronto, ON: University of Toronto Press; 1992.
6. Singh MM, Agarwal RK. Breaking bad news in clinical setting: a systematic review. Ind J Appl Res. 2017;7(12):29–32.
7. Annas G. Informed consent, cancer, and truth in prognosis. N Engl J Med. 1994;330:223–5.
8. Appelbaum PS. Assessment of patients' competence to consent to treatment. N Engl J Med. 2007;357:1834–40.
9. Palmer BW, Dunn LB, Appelbaum PS, Jeste DV. Correlates of treatment-related decision-making capacity among middle-aged and older patients with schizophrenia. Arch Gen Psychiatry. 2004;61:230–6.
10. Palmer BW, Savla GN. The association of specific neuropsychological deficits with capacity to consent to research or treatment. J Int Neuropsychol Soc. 2007;13:1047–59.
11. Grisso T, Appelbaum PS. Assessing competence to consent to treatment: a guide for physicians and other health professionals. New York, NY: Oxford University Press; 1998.
12. Carpenter WT, Gold JM, Lahti AC, Queern CA, Conley RR, Bartko JJ, et al. Decisional capacity for informed consent in schizophrenia research. Arch Gen Psychiatry. 2000;57:533–8.
13. Jeste DV, Depp CA, Palmer BW. Magnitude of impairment in decisional capacity in people with schizophrenia compared to normal subjects: an overview. Schizophr Bull. 2006;32(1):121–8.
14. Kovnick JA, Appelbaum PS, Hoge SK, Leadbetter RA. Competence to consent to research among long-stay inpatients with chronic schizophrenia. Psychiatr Serv. 2003;54(9):1247–52.
15. Moser DJ, Schultz SK, Arndt S, Benjamin ML, Fleming FW, Brems CS, et al. Capacity to provide informed consent for participation in schizophrenia and HIV research. Am J Psychiatry. 2002;159:1201–7.
16. Appelbaum PS. Decisional capacity of patients with schizophrenia to consent to research: taking stock. Schizophr Bull. 2006;32(1):22–5.
17. Dunn LB. Capacity to consent to research in schizophrenia: the expanding evidence base. Behav Sci Law. 2006;24(4):431–45.
18. Palmer BW, Jeste DV. Relationship of individual cognitive abilities to specific components of decisional capacity among middle-aged and older patients with schizophrenia. Schizophr Bull. 2006;32(1):98–106.
19. Lepping P, Stanly T, Turner J. Systematic review on the prevalence of lack of capacity in medical and psychiatric settings. Clin Med. 2015;15(4):337–43.
20. Candia PC, Barba AC. Mental capacity and consent to treatment in psychiatric patients. Curr Opin Psychiatry. 2011;24(5):442–6.
21. Owen GS, Szmukler G, Richardson G, David AS, Raymont V, Freyenhagen F, et al. Decision-making capacity for treatment in psychiatric and medical in-patients: cross-sectional, comparative study. Br J Psychiatry. 2013;203(6):461–7.
22. Raymont V, Bingley W, Buchanan A, David AS, Hayward P, Wessely S, et al. Prevalence of mental incapacity in medical inpatients and associated risk factors: cross-sectional study. Lancet. 2004;364(9443):1421–7.
23. Aydin Er R, Sehiralti M, Aker AT. Preliminary Turkish study of psychiatric in-patients' competence to make treatment decisions. Asia Pac Psychiatry. 2013;5(1):E9–E18.
24. Mandarelli G, Tarsitani L, Parmigiani G, Polselli GM, Frati P, Biondi M, et al. Mental capacity in patients involuntarily or voluntarily receiving psychiatric treatment for an acute mental disorder. J Forensic Sci. 2014;59(4):1002–7.
25. Howe V, Foister K, Jenkins K, Skene L, Copolov D, Keks N. Competence to give informed consent in acute psychosis is associated with symptoms rather than diagnosis. Schizophr Res. 2005;77(2–3):211–4.
26. Cairns R, Maddock C, Buchanan A, David AS, Hayward P, Richardson G, et al. Prevalence and predictors of mental incapacity in psychiatric in-patients. Br J Psychiatry. 2005;187:379–85.
27. Owen GS, David AS, Richardson G, Szmukler G, Hayward P, Hotopf M. Mental capacity, diagnosis and insight in psychiatric in-patients: a cross-sectional study. Psychol Med. 2008;39(8):1389.

28. Parmigiani G, Mandarelli G, Dacquino C, Pompili P, Lelli Chiesa G, Ferracuti S. Decisional capacity to consent to clinical research involving placebo in psychiatric patients. J Forensic Sci. 2016;61(2):388–93.
29. Mandarelli G, Parmigiani G, Tarsitani L, Frati P, Biondi M, Ferracuti S. The relationship between executive functions and capacity to consent to treatment in acute psychiatric hospitalization. J Empir Res Hum Res Ethics. 2012;7(5):63–70.
30. Jeste DV, Palmer BW, Appelbaum PS, Golshan S, Glorioso D, Dunn LB, et al. A new brief instrument for assessing decisional capacity for clinical research. Arch Gen Psychiatry. 2007;64(8):966–74.
31. Barch DM, Ceaser A. Cognition in schizophrenia: core psychological and neural mechanisms. Trends Cogn Sci. 2012;16(1):27–34.
32. Mesholam-Gately RI, Giuliano AJ, Goff KP, Faraone SV, Seidman LJ. Neurocognition in first-episode schizophrenia: a meta-analytic review. Neuropsychology. 2009;23(3):315–36.
33. Hellvin T, Sundet K, Simonsen C, Aminoff SR, Lagerberg TV, Andreassen OA, et al. Neurocognitive functioning in patients recently diagnosed with bipolar disorder. Bipolar Disord. 2012;14(3):227–38.
34. Koren D, Poyurovsky M, Seidman LJ, Goldsmith M, Wenger S, Klein EM. The neuropsychological basis of competence to consent in first-episode schizophrenia: a pilot metacognitive study. Biol Psychiatry. 2005;57(6):609–16.
35. Goldstein G. Neuropsychological heterogeneity in schizophrenia: a consideration of abstraction and problem-solving abilities. Arch Clin Neuropsychol. 1990;5(3):251–64.
36. Holzer JC, Gansler DA, Moczynski NP, Folstein MF. Cognitive functions in the informed consent evaluation process: a pilot study. J Am Acad Psychiatry Law. 1997;25(4):531–40.
37. Schillerstrom JE, Rickenbacker D, Joshi KG, Royall DR. Executive function and capacity to consent to a noninvasive research protocol. Am J Geriatr Psychiatry. 2007;15(2):159–62.
38. Royall DR, Mahurin RK, Gray KF. Bedside assessment of executive cognitive impairment: the executive interview. J Am Geriatr Soc. 1992;40(12):1221–6.
39. Okai D, Owen G, McGuire H, Singh S, Churchill R, Hotopf M. Mental capacity in psychiatric patients: systematic review. Br J Psychiatry. 2007;191(4):291–7.
40. Bellhouse J, Holland AJ, Clare ICH, Gunn M, Watson P. Capacity-based mental health legislation and its impact on clinical practice: 1) admission to hospital. J Ment Health Law. 2013;1:24–37.
41. Bellhouse J, Holland AJ, Clare ICH, Gunn M, Watson P. Capacity-based mental health legislation and its impact on clinical practice: 1) admission to hospital. J Ment Health Law. 2013;1:9–23.
42. Owen GS, Richardson G, David AS, Szmukler G, Hayward P, Hotopf M. Mental capacity to make decisions on treatment in people admitted to psychiatric hospitals: cross sectional study. BMJ. 2008;337:a448.
43. Poythress NG, Cascardi M, Ritterband L. Capacity to consent to voluntary hospitalization: searching for a satisfactory Zinermon screen. Bull Am Acad Psychiatry Law. 1996;24(4):439–52.
44. Appelbaum BC, Appelbaum PS, Grisso T. Competence to consent to voluntary psychiatric hospitalization: a test of a standard proposed by APA. Psychiatr Serv. 1998;49(9):1193–6.
45. Appelbaum PS, Grisso T. Assessing patients' capacities to consent to treatment. N Engl J Med. 1988;319(25):1635–8.
46. Rutledge E, Kennedy M, O'Neill H, Kennedy HG. Functional mental capacity is not independent of the severity of psychosis. Int J Law Psychiatry. 2008;31(1):9–18.
47. Mandarelli G, Carabellese F, Parmigiani G, Bernardini F, Pauselli L, Quartesan R, et al. Treatment decision-making capacity in non-consensual psychiatric treatment: a multicentre study. Epidemiol Psychiatr Sci. 2018;27(5):492–9.
48. Palmer BW, Dunn LB, Depp CA, Eyler LT, Jeste DV. Decisional capacity to consent to research among patients with bipolar disorder: comparison with schizophrenia patients and healthy subjects. J Clin Psychiatry. 2007;68:689–96.

49. Gardner W, Lidz CW, Hoge SK, Monahan J, Eisenberg MM, Bennett NS, et al. Patients' revisions of their beliefs about the need for hospitalization. Am J Psychiatry. 1999;156:1385–91.
50. Bindman J, Reid Y, Szmukler G, Tiller J, Thornicroft G, Leese M. Perceived coercion at admission to psychiatric hospital and engagement with follow-up--a cohort study. Soc Psychiatry Psychiatr Epidemiol. 2005;40(2):160–6.
51. Hiday VA, Swartz MS, Swanson J, Wagner HR. Patient perceptions of coercion in mental hospital admission. Int J Law Psychiatry. 1997;20(2):227–41.
52. Iversen KI, Høyer G, Sexton H, Grønli OK. Perceived coercion among patients admitted to acute wards in Norway. Nord J Psychiatry. 2002;56(6):433–9.
53. Kaltiala-Heino R, Laippala P, Salokangas RKR. Impact of coercion on treatment outcome. Int J Law Psychiatry. 1997;20(3):311–22.
54. Steinert T, Lepping P, Bernhardsgrütter R, Conca A, Hatling T, Janssen W, et al. Incidence of seclusion and restraint in psychiatric hospitals: a literature review and survey of international trends. Soc Psychiatry Psychiatr Epidemiol. 2010;45(9):889–97.
55. Anestis A, Daffern M, Thomas SDM, Podubinski T, Hollander Y, Lee S, et al. Predictors of perceived coercion in patients admitted for psychiatric hospitalization and the stability of these perceptions over time. Psychiatry Psychol Law. 2013;20(4):492–503.
56. Fiorillo A, Giacco D, De Rosa C, Kallert T, Katsakou C, Onchev G, et al. Patient characteristics and symptoms associated with perceived coercion during hospital treatment. Acta Psychiatr Scand. 2012;125(6):460–7.
57. O'Donoghue B, Lyne J, Hill M, O'Rourke L, Daly S, Larkin C, et al. Perceptions of involuntary admission and risk of subsequent readmission at one-year follow-up: the influence of insight and recovery style. J Ment Health. 2011;20(3):249–59.
58. Kjellin L, Høyer G, Engberg M, Kaltiala-Heino R, Sigurjónsdóttir M. Differences in perceived coercion at admission to psychiatric hospitals in the Nordic countries. Soc Psychiatry Psychiatr Epidemiol. 2006;41(3):241–7.
59. Poythress NG, Petrila J, McGaha A, Boothroyd R. Perceived coercion and procedural justice in the Broward mental health court. Int J Law Psychiatry. 2002;25:517–33.
60. NICE. Violence and aggression. Short-term management in mental health, health and community settings. Updated edition. London: NICE; 2015.
61. Fiorillo A, De Rosa C, Del Vecchio V, Jurjanz L, Schnall K, Onchev G, et al. How to improve clinical practice on involuntary hospital admissions of psychiatric patients: suggestions from the EUNOMIA study. Eur Psychiatry. 2011;26(4):201–7.
62. Gardner W, Hoge SK, Bennett N, Roth LH, Lidz CW, Morrahan J, et al. Two scales for measuring patients' perceptions for coercion during mental hospital admission. Behav Sci Law. 1993;11:307–21.
63. Mandarelli G, Parmigiani G, Trobia F, Tessari G, Roma P, Biondi M, et al. The Admission Experience Survey Italian Version (I-AES): a factor analytic study on a sample of 156 acute psychiatric in-patients. Int J Law Psychiatry. 2019;62:111–6.
64. Svindseth MF, Dahl AA, Hatling T. Patients' experience of humiliation in the admission process to acute psychiatric wards. Nord J Psychiatry. 2007;61(1):47–53.
65. Fu JC, Chow PP, Lam LC. The experience of admission to psychiatric hospital among Chinese adult patients in Hong Kong. BMC Psychiatry. 2008;8:86.
66. Gowda GS, Noorthoorn EO, Kumar CN, Nanjegowda RB, Math SB. Clinical correlates and predictors of perceived coercion among psychiatric inpatients: a prospective pilot study. Asian J Psychiatr. 2016;22:34–40.
67. Kjellin L, Andersson K, Bartholdson E, Candefjord IL, Holmstrom H, Jacobsson L, et al. Coercion in psychiatric care – patients' and relatives' experiences from four Swedish psychiatric services. Nord J Psychiatry. 2004;58(2):153–9.
68. De Girolamo G, Barbato A, Bracco R, Gaddini A, Miglio R, Morosini P, et al. Characteristics and activities of acute psychiatric in-patient facilities: national survey in Italy. Br J Psychiatry. 2007;191:170–7.
69. Amaddeo F, Barbui C, Tansella M. State of psychiatry in Italy 35 years after psychiatric reform. A critical appraisal of national and local data. Int Rev Psychiatry. 2012;24(4):314–20.

70. de Girolamo G, Cozza M. The Italian psychiatric reform. A 20-year perspective. Int J Law Psychiatry. 2000;23(3–4):197–214.
71. Sheridan Rains L, Zenina T, Dias MC, Jones R, Jeffreys S, Branthonne-Foster S, et al. Variations in patterns of involuntary hospitalisation and in legal frameworks: an international comparative study. Lancet Psychiatry. 2019;6(5):403–17.
72. Salize HJ, Dressing H. Epidemiology of involuntary placement of mentally ill people across the European Union. Br J Psychiatry. 2004;184:163–8.
73. Dressing H, Salize HJ. Compulsory admission of mentally ill patients in European Union Member States. Soc Psychiatry Psychiatr Epidemiol. 2004;39(10):797–803.
74. Zinkler M, Priebe S. Detention of the mentally ill in Europe--a review. Acta Psychiatr Scand. 2002;106(1):3–8.
75. Cunningham G. Analysis of episodes of involuntary re-admission in Ireland (2007–2010). Ir J Psychol Med. 2012;29(3):180–4.
76. Ng XT, Kelly BD. Voluntary and involuntary care: three-year study of demographic and diagnostic admission statistics at an inner-city adult psychiatry unit. Int J Law Psychiatry. 2012;35(4):317–26.
77. van der Post L, Visch I, Mulder C, Schoevers R, Dekker J, Beekman A. Factors associated with higher risks of emergency compulsory admission for immigrants: a report from the ASAP study. Int J Soc Psychiatry. 2012;58(4):374–80.
78. Hustoft K, Larsen TK, Auestad B, Joa I, Johannessen JO, Ruud T. Predictors of involuntary hospitalizations to acute psychiatry. Int J Law Psychiatry. 2013;36(2):136–43.
79. Wheeler A, Robinson E, Robinson G. Admissions to acute psychiatric inpatient services in Auckland, New Zealand: a demographic and diagnostic review. N Z Med J. 2005;118(1226):U1752.
80. Webber M, Huxley P. Social exclusion and risk of emergency compulsory admission. A case-control study. Soc Psychiatry Psychiatr Epidemiol. 2004;39(12):1000–9.
81. Kelly BD, Clarke M, Browne S, McTigue O, Kamali M, Gervin M, et al. Clinical predictors of admission status in first episode schizophrenia. Eur Psychiatry. 2004;19(2):67–71.
82. Preti A, Rucci P, Santone G, Picardi A, Miglio R, Bracco R, et al. Patterns of admission to acute psychiatric in-patient facilities: a national survey in Italy. Psychol Med. 2009;39(3):485–96.
83. Ministero della Salute. Rapporto salute mentale. Analisi dei dati del sistema informativo per la salute mentale (SISM) Anno. Roma: Ministero della salute; 2016. http://www.salute.gov.it/imgs/C_17_pubblicazioni_2731_allegato.pdf. Accessed 20 December 2019.
84. Gaddini A, Ascoli M, Biscaglia L. Mental health care in Rome. Eur Psychiatry. 2005;20:S294–S7.
85. Canova Mosele PH, Chervenski Figueira G, Antonio Bertuol Filho A, de Lima JAR F, Calegaro VC. Involuntary psychiatric hospitalization and its relationship to psychopathology and aggression. Psychiatry Res. 2018;265:13–8.
86. Montemagni C, Bada A, Castagna F, Frieri T, Rocca G, Scalese M, et al. Predictors of compulsory admission in schizophrenia-spectrum patients: excitement, insight, emotion perception. Prog Neuropsychopharmacol Biol Psychiatry. 2011;35(1):137–45.
87. Berg JW, Appelbaum PS, Lidz CW, Parker L. Informed consent: legal theory and clinical practice. 2nd ed. New York, NY: Oxford University Press; 2001.
88. Dunn LB, Jeste DV. Enhancing informed consent for research and treatment. Neuropsychopharmacology. 2001;24(6):595–607.
89. Appelbaum PS. Consent in impaired populations. Curr Neurol Neurosci Rep. 2010;10(5):367–73.
90. Hostiuc S, Rusu MC, Negoi I, Drima E. Testing decision-making competency of schizophrenia participants in clinical trials. A meta-analysis and meta-regression. BMC Psychiatry. 2018;18(1):2.
91. Wang X, Yu X, Appelbaum PS, Tang H, Yao G, Si T, et al. Longitudinal informed consent competency in stable community patients with schizophrenia: a one-week training and one-year follow-up study. Schizophr Res. 2016;170(1):162–7.

92. Moser DJ, Reese RL, Hey CT, Schultz SK, Arndt S, Beglinger LJ, et al. Using a brief intervention to improve decisional capacity in schizophrenia research. Schizophr Bull. 2006;32(1):116–20.
93. Palmer BW, Harmell AL, Dunn LB, Kim SY, Pinto LL, Golshan S, et al. Multimedia aided consent for Alzheimer's disease research. Clin Gerontol. 2018;41(1):20–32.
94. Mittal D, Palmer BW, Dunn LB, Landes R, Ghormley C, Beck C, et al. Comparison of two enhanced consent procedures for patients with Mild Alzheimer Disease or Mild Cognitive Impairment. Am J Geriatr Psychiatry. 2007;15(2):163–7.
95. Rubright J, Sankar P, Casarett DJ, Gur R, Xie SX, Karlawish J. A memory and organizational aid improves Alzheimer disease research consent capacity: results of a randomized, controlled trial. Am J Geriatr Psychiatry. 2010;18(12):1124–32.

Post-aggression Debrief

8

Marta Caminiti, Riccardo Di Febo, and Mauro Pallagrosi

8.1   Introduction

Episodes of violence and aggression in mental health settings occur most frequently in psychiatric inpatient units. De-escalation methods, like those presented in this book, are essential tools in order to prevent and minimize the occurrence of such episodes. However, it is not possible to reduce to zero the risk of adverse events, and aggressions towards staff and use of restraint measures remain a not negligible part of the work of the psychiatric wards.

The manifestation of violence and aggression depends on a combination of intrinsic factors, such as personality characteristics and psychopathological condition of the patients, and extrinsic factors, such as the attitudes and behaviours of surrounding staff and the physical and structural setting of the psychiatric wards [1]. According to scientific literature, the most significant intrinsic factors associated with and predictive of violent behaviour are poor compliance to psychopharmacological treatment, compulsory and protracted periods of hospitalization and history of previous aggressive episodes [2–4].

The impact of violence and aggression is significant and manifold, adversely affecting health and safety of both service users and staff members. In Italy, for example, since the acute inpatient wards are usually not provided with seclusion rooms, these episodes are mostly followed by pharmacological or mechanical restraint measures, which have consequences in themselves.

In other countries, the practice of post-aggression debrief, which is considered a tertiary prevention strategy, has become a fundamental part of multidimensional programs of intervention such as, for example, "The Six Core Strategies for Reducing Seclusion and Restraint Use" proposed by Huckshorn and adopted in American psychiatric units (6CS).

M. Caminiti · R. Di Febo · M. Pallagrosi (✉)
Department of Human Neuroscience, Sapienza University of Rome, Rome, Italy
e-mail: mauro.pallagrosi@uniroma1.it

© Springer Nature Switzerland AG 2021   133
M. Biondi et al. (eds.), *Empathy, Normalization and De-escalation*,
https://doi.org/10.1007/978-3-030-65106-0_8

The focus of this chapter is indeed the post-aggression debrief, which is as a practice of reviewing an aggressive event in order to process the experience and to learn from it. Debriefing aims at addressing the emotional impact of aggression and its consequences on the people involved (both service users and staff) and at analysing each incident in order to identify practice issues and organizational and system problems and ultimately to prevent recurrences.

It will be described how post-aggression debrief was developed, from its first application in non-medical settings to its current use in psychiatric wards.

Some practical guidelines will be provided about the modalities for conducting post-aggression debrief for both patients and healthcare professionals, according to the latest studies and the authors' clinical experience. Debrief will be presented as a tool for fostering a better working climate among staff members and reducing the stress and the emotional turmoil associated with an aggressive episode.

Finally, post-aggression debrief will be discussed for its role as a way to give significance to aggressive events in terms of possible shared meaning between the patient and the staff. In other words, debriefing will be presented as a chance to comprehend the patient's psychopathological world, to restore a narrative coherence beyond the traumatic and violent event and to keep a safe and trustable therapeutic environment.

8.2   Debriefing: Definition and Historical Background

Debriefing is defined as "the practice of reviewing an event, in order to process aspects of the experience and learn from it" [5]. It takes place following a critical event or a difficult task that has been completed: this practice is structured as a meeting between staff members, led and coordinated by a designated facilitator that encourages staff to reflect on their actions in order to develop knowledge and skills. During debriefing, team members discuss what happened, what has been done and what strategies should be better adopted in the future.

Over time, debriefing has been used in different operational contexts and in different forms, fostering a culture of sharing, openness to change and willingness to learn from past experience.

The first documented attempt at debriefing took place in a military setting during World War II. During his service as chief combat historian for the US army, L.A. Marshall was known for gathering his troops to engage them in post-combat reviews. Marshall used to encourage soldiers to share their experience and to rigorously reconstruct the dynamics of combat. Having this space to reflect on the events that had just occurred was instrumental for improving both their performance on the field and their cohesion as a group [6].

Gradually, debriefing begins to be used as a practice of returning to a critical event, providing emotional support to people exposed to a potentially traumatic episode. During the Vietnam War, military psychiatrists began promoting post-battle meetings to analyse soldiers' emotional responses and to support their combat stress. The purpose of this form of debriefing was to allow soldiers to externalize thoughts, memories and emotions related to a potential traumatic experience in order to understand and normalize them [6, 7].

The first form of psychological debriefing was developed by Jeffrey T. Mitchell, Professor of Emergency Health Services at the University of Maryland, to mitigate the emotional impact on staff involved in traumatic situations and facilitate normal recovery processes [8]. Mitchell's debriefing model, called *Critical Incident Stress Debriefing* (CISD), was originally an operational protocol intended for ambulance staff and was later extended to a "crisis support programme" for police officers, firefighters, prisoners of war and people exposed to natural disasters. The CISD is a group meeting led by a debriefer who encourages people to express their feelings and reactions related to a traumatic event. Debriefing after trauma helped individuals to overcome their overwhelming emotions, such sense of helplessness and guilt: the act of reliving the episode as a group allowed subjects to feel safe and recreate a sense of order and trust among them [6].

During the 1980s, debriefing techniques began to be used to improve the quality of medical services, hospital staff skills, critical event management and the organization of health services. The first form of technical debriefing was implemented by David M. Gaba, a clinician-educator anaesthesiologist at the Veterans Affairs Palo Alto Health Care System, who devised a structured training practice for anaesthesiologists. This new form of debriefing consisted in the simulation of a critical event, aimed at training anaesthesiologists in the management of complex clinical situations: the entire process was supervised by a facilitator, who systematically provided feedback [9]. Following the experience of Dr. Gaba, debriefing has been progressively adopted for training specialists from different medical disciplines [10].

Over the years, debriefing potential of application in the mental health field became more and more evident: debrief started to be introduced as a tool for reviewing critical events occurring in the management of difficult cases, especially in psychiatric inpatient units.

8.3   Post-aggression Debrief in Mental Health

Violence and aggression are common in psychiatric inpatients units. Aggressive behaviours can endanger the safety of the psychiatric ward and may lead to serious physical and psychological consequences for both patients and staff. Violence can take different forms: verbal and physical threats, attacks on objects or people and self-directed conducts, such as self-harm.

Aggressive behaviour can be contained through different kinds of intervention: relational, pharmacological and, in critical situations, physical, such as restraint, which can be emotionally challenging for everyone involved. The way the staff interacts with patients and with each other can play an important role: a study aimed at estimating the effects of team processes on nurse decision-making on seclusion showed a correlation between the team reflexivity (defined by Dr. West as: "the extent to which group members overly reflect upon, and communicate about, the group's objectives, strategies and processes and adapt them to current or anticipated circumstances") and its tendency to avoid coercive practices. Moreover, it showed that the use of restraint was determined more by team characteristics (such as staffing level and confidence in each other within the team) and interpersonal factors (like the patient's approachability) than by the patient's individual characteristics (diagnosis, history of seclusion, severity of the threat, target of the threat) [11].

Restriction has been described by service users as a distressing event that had the power to reawaken previous traumatic memories. Feelings of fear, anger and abandonment are common among restricted patients. Moreover, they experience restriction as punitive, reporting failure to have their basic needs met, an inadequate communication with care providers and the absence of an adequate post-aggression follow-up. After the application of containment measures, patients can feel isolated and ashamed, especially when not involved in a post-aggression review [12–16].

Restraint measures induce negative emotions even in the health staff such as anxiety, fear, anger, frustration, distress and feeling conflicted [17]. Healthcare providers often do not find an opportunity to reflect and express their negative emotions after an event of aggression and restraint. This situation can have negative impact on staff, their relationship with the patient and the organization of services, increasing the risk of aggression in psychiatry wards [18].

Because of its complex and multifaceted nature, aggressive behaviour requires an emotional, technical and organizational effort by health staff in order to find better strategies and to improve quality of care. After analysing multiple reviews on the topic of post-seclusion/restraint (S/R), Ph.D. Marie Hélène Goulet proceeded to define post-aggression debrief as "a complex intervention, taking place after a seclusion/restraint episode and targeting the patient and healthcare team to enhance the care experience and provide meaningful learning for the patient, staff, and organization". The National Institute for Health and Care Excellence (NICE) guidelines recommend to conduct a post-incident debrief in inpatient psychiatric settings, in order to identify and address ongoing risks and any physical or emotional harm to service users or staff. NICE considers debrief a useful tool for its potential to anticipate and reduce episodes of behavioural escalation, promote changes in care practices and create a space of mutual understanding and empathy [1, 19].

Post-aggression debrief should explore the triggers involved in the aggression (patient symptoms, environments, type of relationship between staff and patient, coping strategies used), engaging both the patients and the care providers in discussing what happened, why the restraining measures were used and how they feel about it [1]. This procedure prompts a reflective attitude in everyone involved and fosters mutual learning and changes in practice. Also, it correlates with a significant reduction in the number of violent events and duration spent in seclusion and restraint in the intervention wards: this improves the quality of care as well as the safety of the ward [5, 19].

In 2014, Te Pou, a national centre of evidence-based workforce development for mental health in New Zealand, commissioned a summary of relevant literature about debriefing following seclusion and restraint and found that debriefing is often reported as being one of multiple strategies that can be used in combination to successfully reduce seclusion and/or restraint [5]. For example, post-aggression debriefing is a fundamental part of "The Six Core Strategies for Reducing Seclusion and Restraint Use" (6CS), proposed by Huckshorn and adopted in American psychiatric units. The application in eight US states of the 6CS program showed an average reduction of the overall secluded population, the overall amount of seclusion hours and the percentage of patients who were restrained equal to, respectively, 17%, 19% and 30% [20].

Despite there being several studies supporting the effectiveness of post-aggression debrief as part of an integrated programme of intervention in reducing restraint in psychiatric units, there is limited evidence regarding its impact as a single intervention. However, the 2013 research that Whitecross undertook in Melbourne, comparing a group of patients who received a post-incident debriefing after restraint with a control group being offered the usual care, did show that post-aggression debrief reduced restraint hours in psychiatric units [21].

When it comes to the impact of debriefing in reducing negative emotions related to restriction, the results are controversial. According to a study conducted by Jacobowitz, an associate professor of Adelphi University in New York, debriefing may facilitate the development of resilience in nurses with respect to the risk of PTSD [22]. On the contrary, Whitecross' study showed that post-aggression debrief did not improve symptoms of post-traumatic stress due to containment, compared to the control group [21]; similar conclusions have been reached by other studies [23–25].

Overall, two forms of post-aggression debrief have been described: one focused on the health staff and one focused on the patient [5, 26]. *Staff debriefing* is a rigorous event analysis to identify system problems and prevent recurrences. Also, it's an experiential learning opportunity by facilitating better problem management through shared treatment plans. *Patient-focused debriefing* encourages the patient to reflect on his dysfunctional behaviour and emotion and find new strategies and shared solutions to avoid recurrence of violent behaviour. In addition, it is a useful device for clinicians to understand the patient's perspective restoring an atmosphere of trust between clinicians and patients.

8.3.1 Staff-Focused Post-aggression Debrief

8.3.1.1 Summary of Evidence

Post-aggression debriefing can be a very useful tool not only for patients but also for the hospital staff. The main goal remains a significant reduction in the number of events and time spent in seclusion and restraint in the intervention ward, but other important goals are also achievable.

Psychiatrists and nurses can gather and discuss a violent event that has occurred during seclusion which can have several beneficial effects: to ensure the staff safety, to officially document the event, to enhance mental coping, to prevent stress reactions and to identify who is in need of further professional intervention [5, 27]. Also, debrief can accomplish a quality improvement of care and an organizational development among the staff [5].

Debriefing has a positive impact on the staff: it improves staff cohesion, reinforcing a supportive behaviour between colleagues, especially after a potentially distressing event [19, 28]. A properly conducted debrief can improve individual and team performance by approximately 20–25% [29].

In the last decade, many international studies and reviews have been released on debriefing, and in 2017, NICE has published specific guidelines for conducting an effective post-aggression staff debrief. In this paragraph, it will be discussed who should participate, what is the appropriate time frame, how to lead a debriefing and what should be explored during this process, according to literature.

8.3.1.2 Participants

Psychiatrists, nurses and every member of the psychiatric ward staff who was involved in any event that featured the use of a restrictive intervention to manage violence or aggression (restraint, rapid tranquillization or seclusion) should be involved in post-aggression debriefing [1].

Executive level committees (head physician, head nurse and supervisors) can be part of the debriefing group, with two main purposes: (a) to support the treatment team by providing expertise in addressing the behavioural and support needs of particular service users and (b) to provide administrative level support for quality improvement and broader systems change for seclusion and restraint reduction [5].

8.3.1.3 Time Frame

Post-aggression debrief usually takes place a few hours to 72 h post-event, depending on the availability of the staff and the time for reflection they consider appropriate, because "sometimes, when you're full of adrenaline, it's hard to really talk about what you experienced" [19].

According to the 2014 review of Te Pou, the debrief can take place in three different sessions:

1. **Immediate post-aggression debrief**, as soon as possible after the event. The goal is to officially document the event while information about the incident is fresh, ensure the safety of the staff and help as an immediate stress relief. It provides evidence that can support future meaningful plan revisions.
2. **Formal post-aggression debrief**: this process takes place a few days later and includes rigorous methods of analysis and problem-solving in relation to the event, addressing staff emotions and thoughts;
3. **Executive post-aggression debrief** that might occur fortnightly to monthly depending on the number of incidents and urgency: the aim is using staff and service user debriefing information in order to make concrete changes on the psychiatric ward organization [5].

The three forms of staff-focused post-aggression debrief are summarized in Fig. 8.1.

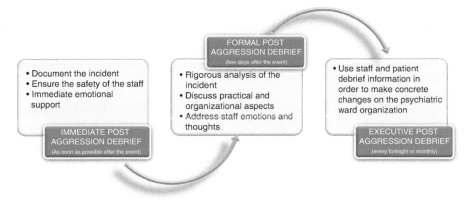

Fig. 8.1 Forms of staff-focused post-aggression debrief [5]

8.3.1.4 How to Lead a Debriefing

Post-aggression debrief can be self-led or led by a facilitator.

A self-led debrief can be effective when participants have enough ability to reflect and criticize by themselves. It might be more appropriate for experienced healthcare professionals rather than less practiced ones, due to a gap in knowledge and problem-solving skills between them.

Facilitator-led debrief allows participants to reflect on their performance in a psychologically protected environment: having a small group of participants can help the facilitator to create a safe sharing environment where workers can share more of their feelings and reactions [30, 31].

Leading a debriefing is not a simple task. Specific training for members of the staff, interested in becoming a facilitator, has been proposed. An interesting example of training, in a general medical setting, is provided by a recent experience from Michigan Medical School, where a 2-h workshop was organized for senior residents to provide them with the knowledge and skills to lead debriefing sessions within their teams [32]. The survey, pre- and post-workshop, reported a significant increase in resident comfort and appreciation about leading a debriefing session, as well as in recognition of personal distress. However, in psychiatric setting, due to the complexity of the clinical situations, facilitators are usually identified with senior clinical representatives from the inpatient service.

8.3.1.5 Debriefing Technique

Post-aggression debrief is a rigorous event analysis of each incident to address system problems and prevent recurrences [5]. It should take place in a private area, where it is possible to have face-to-face meetings [19]. Staff can use information from the patient's post-aggression debrief, in order to be fully aware of the point of view of the other parts involved [5].

To gain maximum results, it is important to ensure alignment between participants, focus and intent [29]. It is necessary to instil with participants the importance of being open, constructive and without judgment, in order to create a respectful atmosphere and don't let a specific staff member feel targeted [19].

Studies reporting the use of formal staff debriefing described the importance of applying *root cause analysis* (RCA), a structured process for deeper problem-solving. The advantage of RCA is that it encourages staff to take a no-blame approach, as the analysis concerns setting, situation and system rather than treatment or care provided by an individual [5].

During debriefing, it is crucial to focus on what caused the break point in the relationship between the patient and the staff. It is appropriate to encourage participants to engage a constructive re-enactment of the sequence of actions that led the events to an escalation.

Debriefing can also be the appropriate setting for an accurate evaluation of the use of protocols for seclusion and restraint, assessing whether the staff was coordinated, effective and respectful during the procedure. Collecting feedback from doctors and nurses can become an opportunity to make adjustments on the protocols that must be adopted in these circumstances, in order to guarantee the safety of both patients and operators.

Facilitators can use post-aggression debrief as an instrument to detect which members of the staff need more help processing the trauma and to whom it can be offered additional assistance after the event. Debriefing can be the first step to create a support system between co-workers that make them feel less alone and overwhelmed [27].

According to literature, it is recommended to conduct debriefing using a structured sequence of questions that are listed in Fig. 8.2 [1, 19].

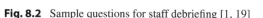

ENVIRONMENT
- What was the environment like?
- Do we know if the patient had been S/R before?
- Did a member of the team develop a trusting relationship with the patient?
- Did we know the patient well enough to identify his or her personal triggers?
- Did the patient's behavior change during or before the shift?
- Did someone in the team speak to the patient before the incident?

EARLY IDENTIFICATION OF BEHAVIORAL CHANGE
- When did we respond to changes in behavior?
- Where there any signs or warnings that the patient was upset?
- What were the first verbal and nonverbal signs?

TRIGGERS AND CONFLICT
- What were the triggers for the patient's aggressive or dangerous?
- Could the trigger for conflict (symptoms, personal, environment) have been prevented?

LENGTH OF S/R
- What were the criteria for releasing the patient and were they appropriate?
- Could the patient have come out of S/R earlier?

INTERVENTIONS ATTEMPTED TO S/R
- What intervention was attempted before and why?
- Was the intervention delayed for some reason?
- How did the patient respond to the intervention?
- Was staff prepared to intervene at the moment?
- What have been attempted but was not and why?

REASON FOR THE DECISION TO USE S/R
- What was the exact behavior justyifing S/R?
- What would have happened if there had been no S/R?
- Why was this decision taken?

APPLICATION OF S/R
- Where the principles of the protocol met??
- Did staff order S/R only in response to imminent danger?
- Was S/R applied safely?

LEARNING FROM THE S/R
- What can we learn from this S/R episode in terms of the patient's treatment plan and our practice?

Fig. 8.2 Sample questions for staff debriefing [1, 19]

8.3.2 Patient-Focused Post-aggression Debrief

8.3.2.1 Summary of Evidence

Patient-focused debrief aims at exploring the patient's perspective of the event, his or her feeling and reaction regarding the violent behaviour and the restraint experience. This process can be described as a "talking therapy that offers the patient the opportunity to make sense of their experience and bring about emotional resolution and healing" [21].

During debriefing, patients and healthcare professionals try to analyse the episode of aggression in order to find shared alternative coping strategies to avoid recurrences.

Patient's active participation is instrumental for him or her to develop personal responsibility, sense of agency and empowerment, which are fundamental elements of the recovery process [33].

According to literature, patients express the desire to debrief after an aggressive event, and they believe that seclusion/restraint experiences could be prevented by talking about the meaning of their feelings before their behaviour escalation [5, 34].

Healthcare staff should inform patients of the possibility of having a debrief after an episode of behavioural escalation and explain how this practice should be performed and its objectives.

It will be discussed who should participate in the patient-focused debrief, what is the appropriate time frame and what should be explored during this process, according to literature.

8.3.2.2 Participants

Patient-focused post-aggression debrief is attended by both healthcare staff members and patients. The health staff includes psychiatrists, nurses and any member directly or indirectly involved in the critical event. Patients may be reluctant to talk to the healthcare professionals directly involved, still experiencing feelings of anger, mistrust and resentment towards them. Hence, it is useful to ask the patient who are the members of the staff that he or she feels most comfortable with, in order to be sure to involve them in the debrief. Members of the staff not directly involved in the violent event can intervene as facilitators, in order to create an atmosphere of trust and therapeutic alliance. Some studies have suggested to involve in the debrief a patient's representative, such as a family member, a support administrator or a trusted person, who may promote the patient's voice and allow the patient to level his/her perceived feeling of powerlessness [5].

8.3.2.3 Time Frame

Post-aggression debrief should take place when the patient feels ready and mentally able to participate. Healthcare professionals should not force the confrontation and should show flexibility to debrief in the more appropriate time frame for the patient. If the debrief takes place too soon, the patient could still have not fully recovered from the experience of containment: this can hurt the patient and affect the outcome of the debriefing, because it is crucial that he or she feels emotionally able to retrace the dynamics of the event and reflect on his or her feelings. On the contrary, a debrief starting too late after the event can increase the patient's feelings of isolation, distress and neglect [5].

8.3.2.4 Debriefing Technique

There are three main components of debrief that help the patients to reflect on their own behaviour and to try to change their dysfunctional reactions: behavioural analysis, education and problem-solving.

Behavioural analysis encourages the patient to examine his or her behavioural responses and the emotions related to the aggressive event. The patient's perspective can be useful for the health staff to understand what could have been done to avoid the outburst of a violent behaviour. A series of questions that can be used in course of behaviour analysis will be provided in Fig. 8.3.

The *education* phase gives the patient the opportunity to understand the reasoning behind containing interventions. In this phase, the medical staff shares with the patient why certain therapeutic choices have been made [5].

Lastly, the phase of *problem-solving* is aimed at finding solutions to the problems which have been identified during behavioural analysis. The staff invite the patient to hypothesize alternative ways to manage intense and chaotic emotional states, stimulating the patient's resources in developing less destructive coping strategies.

The three phases of the patient-focused post-aggression debrief are summarized in Fig. 8.4.

Fig. 8.3 Sample questions for behaviour analysis during patient-focused debriefing [5]

- What happened that led you to be aggressive?
- How did you feel before you got aggressive?
- Did the behavior of a member of the staff made you angry?
- Was there any aspects of the ward environment that made you nervous?
- Have you ever had the same aggressive reaction in the past?
- Have you ever felt the same emotion in the past?
- Have you ever found an alternative way to deal with these negative emotions?
- Was there anything the staff could have done to avoid your aggressive behavior?
- What do you think about your aggressive reaction?
- Is there anything else you want to share that can help us understand how to prevent these episode from happening in the future?

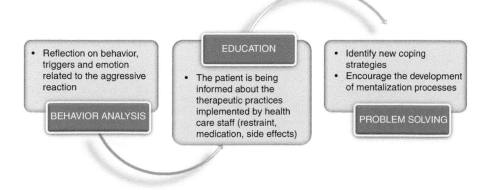

Fig. 8.4 Phases of the patient-focused debriefing [5]

8.4   Discussion

Empirical research has focused on post-aggression debriefing mostly as a part of broader programmes of intervention, like the one presented in this book. However, even if empirical findings are lacking, debriefing by itself can reasonably play a crucial role in improving the quality of clinical practice and reducing aggressive episodes in psychiatric wards [5].

Debriefing should be routinely offered to both patients and staff involved in aggression and restraint episodes. As described above, it can be provided according to different focuses and timing, depending on whether it is thought for the patient or the staff members.

In general, the debriefing process should consist in a rigorous analysis of objective *facts*, followed by an open discussion about subjective feelings, thoughts and suggestions about potential changes in service organization and practice. As written in the Te Pou guidelines, in fact, "Debriefing is future focused as the goal is to prevent problems rather than placing blame for the event that occurred" [5]. For this reason, the possibility to distinguish the concrete behaviours and the contextual factors from the emotions associated with the event is crucial, and the facilitators, when present, should be specifically trained for this ability.

According to the Te Pou guidelines, the main goal of the immediate post-aggression staff debriefing is to give support and to ensure the safety of all persons involved. It should aim at restoring as soon as possible the unit's pre-crisis *milieu*, and it is usually based on the empathic and spontaneous support provided by the staff members not directly involved in the episode. In other words, it represents a sort of groupal reaction, which makes the individual feel belonging to a supportive work team. In our opinion, this phase is of particular importance, as its effectiveness strictly depends on the work environment established by the group through a daily commitment and cannot simply rely on natural attitudes or algorithmic procedures.

At a later time (usually within 48–72 h), a more formal debriefing, based on a documented report of the incident, can provide an important opportunity to analyse facts and emotions, with a double aim: to review the incident, in order to discuss the implied practical and organizational aspects, and, even more importantly, to allow the participants to express and reflect on their emotions and lived experience.

We consider the latter as an essential part of the everyday practice of an acute inpatient wards for two main reasons. On the one hand, the feeling and experience of staff members, when held in a not judgemental atmosphere, can give a valuable contribution to a deeper comprehension of the patient's mental functioning [35]. On the other hand, the capacity of a work group to support, sustain and elaborate complex and often intense negative feelings (i.e. fear, guilt, impotence and shock) can reverberate in the therapeutic atmosphere of the unit. The feasibility of this reflective operation naturally implies the existence of both a solid and respected leadership and an adequate flexibility of the group in terms of cooperative atmosphere and willingness to reflect on its own work.

Indeed, a psychopathologically and psychodynamically oriented perspective on the process of debriefing could help to promote the research of a meaningful comprehension of the violent episodes, integrating the operational approach proposed by the international guidelines. Within this perspective, aggressive behaviours and the resulting restraint measures can be viewed as an indicator of a punctiform failure in communication, where acts take the place of words and shareable thoughts. These episodes, thus, could become the object of a psychopathological reflection, through which it may be possible to restore a sense of meaning, fostering a therapeutic process of mentalization for both staff and patients.

This approach is founded on the assumption that each clinical situation is characterized by peculiarities that could be explored in detail. Just to give an example, with regard to acute delusional patients, aggression can be seen as the only way of expressing unbearable emotional burden, and only experienced staff can deal with these outbursts without feeling deeply affected and becoming reactive. This kind of clinical situations can be retrospectively analysed and discussed from a phenomenological psychopathological point of view, enhancing the possibility of positively managing these otherwise incomprehensible disruptive behaviours in the future. It can be helpful, in fact, to explore patient's experiential structures, such as the inter-subjectivity dimension, in order to link apparently disconnected phenomena together and examine how the patient's delusional scheme may have inglobed staff members during an aggressive episode [36].

Thus, according to this model, staff debriefing should include, together with the aforementioned empathic support and practical issues, a specific psychopathological reflection. This implies that the presence of a facilitator with a specific expertise in psychopathology is generally required. In addition, it seems to us that the possibility of giving sense to "acting out" episodes might contribute also to preserve the work group from negative and potential destructive dynamics. The work in psychiatric inpatient units, in fact, can be a very challenging task, and one of the main protective factors in order to prevent burnout phenomena is to make the staff members feel supported by a well-functioning group.

The patient-focused post-aggression debrief main goal is to heighten the patient's empowerment and to encourage his or her use of more functional solutions for the future. Also regarding the patient-focused post-aggression debrief, our proposal implies an integration of a phenomenological psychopathological perspective about the lived experience of the aggressive episode and the restraint measure taken, from the patient's point of view. The purpose is to rescue, through empathic understanding, the subjective quality and the personal meaning of abnormal phenomena [37]. The focus is on personal identity, self-esteem and self-image of the patient, all aspects that can be potentially damaged by the experience of being restrained after an episode of aggression, when a narration and a possibility of dialogue with the other do not occur. In our clinical experience, this can be a very traumatic experience, especially for young patients at their first admission, and it can bring to potentially serious consequences, in terms of suicidality. The exploration of patient's intentionality, on the other hand, may contribute to restore a sense of agency and temporal self coherence [38], always deeply threatened by mental disorder.

In conclusion, post-aggression debriefing, as a procedural technique possibly integrated with a psychopathological reflection, should be viewed as a valuable tool for clinical practice, since it may transform the aggressive episodes from potentially traumatic experiences into occasions for understanding, rethinking and improving the everyday therapeutic work.

References

1. National Institute for Health and Care Excellence. Overview | Violent and aggressive behaviours in people with mental health problems | Quality standards. London: NICE; 2017. https://www.nice.org.uk/guidance/qs154. Accessed 10 April 2020.
2. Cornaggia CM, Beghi M, Pavone F, Barale F. Aggression in psychiatry wards: a systematic review. Psychiatry Res. 2011;189(1):10–20.
3. Di Lorenzo R, Vecchi L, Artoni C, Mongelli F, Ferri P. Demographic and clinical characteristics of patients involuntarily hospitalized in an italian psychiatric ward: a 1-year retrospective analysis. Acta Biomed. 2018;89(6):17–28.
4. Sato M, Noda T, Sugiyama N, Yoshihama F, Miyake M, Ito H. Characteristics of aggression among psychiatric inpatients by ward type in Japan: using the Staff Observation Aggression Scale – Revised (SOAS-R). Int J Ment Health Nurs. 2017;26(6):602–11.
5. Sutton D, Webster S, Wilson M. Debriefing following seclusion and restraint. 2014. http://www.tepou.co.nz/resources/debriefing-following-seclusion-and-restraint-a-summary-of-relevant-literature/547. Accessed 10 April 2020.
6. Kaplan Z, Iancu I, Bodner E. A review of psychological debriefing after extreme stress. Psychiatr Serv. 2001;52(6):824–7.
7. Solomon Z, Benbenishty R. The role of proximity, immediacy, and expectancy in frontline treatment of combat stress reaction among Israelis in the Lebanon War. Am J Psychiatry. 1986;143(5):613–7.
8. Mitchell J. When disaster strikes … the critical incident stress debriefing process. J Emerg Med Serv. 1983;8:36.
9. Gaba DM, DeAnda A. A comprehensive anesthesia simulation environment: re-creating the operating room for research and training. Anesthesiology. 1988;69(3):387–94.
10. Issenberg SB, McGaghie WC, Petrusa ER, Gordon DL, Scalese RJ. Features and uses of high-fidelity medical simulations that lead to effective learning: a BEME systematic review. Med Teach. 2005;27(1):10–28.
11. Boumans CE, Egger JIM, Souren PM, Mann-PollL PS, Hutschemaekers GJM. Nurses' decision on seclusion: patient characteristics, contextual factors and reflexivity in teams. J Psychiatr Ment Health Nurs. 2012;19(3):264–70.
12. Bonner G, Lowe T, Rawcliffe D, Wellman N. Trauma for all: a pilot study of the subjective experience of physical restraint for mental health inpatients and staff in the UK. J Psychiatr Ment Health Nurs. 2002;9(4):465–73.
13. Donat DC. Special section on seclusion and restraint: encouraging alternatives to seclusion, restraint, and reliance on PRN drugs in a public psychiatric hospital. Psychiatr Serv. 2005;56(9):1105–8.
14. Keski-Valkama A, Koivisto AM, Eronen M, Kaltiala-Heino R. Forensic and general psychiatric patients' view of seclusion: a comparison study. J Forensic Psychiatry Psychol. 2010;21(3):446–61.

15. Kontio R, Joffe G, Putkonen H, Kuosmanen L, Hane K, Holi M, Välimäki M. Seclusion and restraint in psychiatry: patients' experiences and practical suggestions on how to improve practices and use alternatives. Perspect Psychiatr Care. 2012;48(1):16–24.

16. Larue C, Dumais A, Boyer R, Goulet MH, Bonin JP, Baba N. The experience of seclusion and restraint in psychiatric settings: perspectives of patients. Issues Ment Health Nurs. 2013;34(5):317–24.

17. Baroni J. The psychological effects of restraints on mental health workers. 2018. https://aura.antioch.edu/etds. Accessed 10 April 2020.

18. Sequeira H, Halstead S. The psychological effects on nursing staff of administering physical restraint in a secure psychiatric hospital: 'when I go home, it's then that I think about it'. Br J Foren Pract. 2004;6(1):3–15.

19. Goulet MH, Larue C, Lemieux AJ. A pilot study of "post-seclusion and/or restraint review" intervention with patients and staff in a mental health setting. Perspect Psychiatr Care. 2018;54(2):212–20.

20. Wieman DA, Camacho-Gonsalves T, Huckshorn KA, Leff S. Multisite study of an evidence-based practice to reduce seclusion and restraint in psychiatric inpatient facilities. Psychiatr Serv. 2014;65(3):345–51.

21. Whitecross F, Seeary A, Lee S. Measuring the impacts of seclusion on psychiatry inpatients and the effectiveness of a pilot single-session post-seclusion counselling intervention. Int J Ment Health Nurs. 2013;22(6):512–21.

22. Jacobowitz W. PTSD in psychiatric nurses and other mental health providers: a review of the literature. Issues Ment Health Nurs. 2013;34(11):787–95.

23. Arendt M, Elklit A. Effectiveness of psychological debriefing. Acta Psychiatr Scand. 2001;104(6):423–37.

24. Devilly GJ, Wright R, Gist R. A função do debriefing psicológico no tratamento de vítimas de trauma. Rev Bras Psiquiatr. 2003;25(Suppl 1):41–5.

25. Grundlingh H, Knight L, Naker D, Devries K. Secondary distress in violence researchers: a randomised trial of the effectiveness of group debriefings. BMC Psychiatry. 2017;17(1):204.

26. Fisher WA. Elements of successful restraint and seclusion reduction programs and their application in a large, urban, state psychiatric hospital. J Psychiatr Pract. 2003;9(1):7–15.

27. Knobler HY, Nachshoni T, Jaffe E, Peretz G, Yehuda YB. Psychological guidelines for a medical team debriefing after a stressful event. Mil Med. 2007;172(6):581–5.

28. Mangaoil RA, Cleverley K, Peter E. Immediate staff debriefing following seclusion or restraint use in inpatient mental health settings: a scoping review. Clin Nurs Res. 2020;29:479.

29. Tannenbaum SI, Cerasoli CP. Do team and individual debriefs enhance performance? A meta-analysis. Hum Factors. 2013;55(1):231–45.

30. Armstrong K, Zatzick D, Metzler T, Weiss DS, Marmar CR, Garma S, Ronfeldt H, Roepke L. Debriefing of American red cross personnel: pilot study on participants' evaluations and case examples from the 1994 Los Angeles earthquake relief operation. Soc Work Health Care. 1998;27(1):33–50.

31. Kim YJ, Yoo JH. The utilization of debriefing for simulation in healthcare: a literature review. Nurse Educ Pract. 2020;43(January):102698.

32. Govindan M, Keefer P, Sturza J, Stephens M, Malas N. Empowering residents to process distressing events: a debriefing workshop. MedEdPORTAL. 2019;15:10809.

33. Hammervold UE, Norvoll R, Aas RW, Sagvaag H. Post-incident review after restraint in mental health care - a potential for knowledge development, recovery promotion and restraint prevention. A scoping review. BMC Health Serv Res. 2019;19(1):235.

34. Faschingbauer KM, Peden-McAlpine C, Tempel W. Use of seclusion: finding the voice of the patient to influence practice. J Psychosoc Nurs Ment Health Serv. 2013;51(7):32–8.

35. Pallagrosi M, Fonzi L, Picardi A, Biondi M. Association between clinician's subjective experience during patient evaluation and psychiatric diagnosis. Psychopathology. 2016;49(2):83–94. https://doi.org/10.1159/000444506.

36. Parnas J, Zahavi D. The role of phenomenology in psychiatric diagnosis and classification. In: Psychiatric diagnosis and classification. Hoboken, NJ: John Wiley & Sons, Ltd; 2003. p. 137–62.
37. Stanghellini G, Rosfort R. Empathy as a sense of autonomy. Psychopathology. 2013;46(5):337–44.
38. Fuchs T, Pallagrosi M. Phenomenology of temporality and dimensional psychopathology. In: Dimensional psychopathology. Cham: Springer International Publishing; 2018. p. 287–300.